Enida Petro

Early Childhood Caries in Tirana, Albania

Enida Petro

Early Childhood Caries in Tirana, Albania

LAP LAMBERT Academic Publishing

Impressum / Imprint

Bibliografische Information der Deutschen Nationalbibliothek: Die Deutsche Nationalbibliothek verzeichnet diese Publikation in der Deutschen Nationalbibliografie; detaillierte bibliografische Daten sind im Internet über http://dnb.d-nb.de abrufbar.

Alle in diesem Buch genannten Marken und Produktnamen unterliegen warenzeichen-, marken- oder patentrechtlichem Schutz bzw. sind Warenzeichen oder eingetragene Warenzeichen der jeweiligen Inhaber. Die Wiedergabe von Marken, Produktnamen, Gebrauchsnamen, Handelsnamen, Warenbezeichnungen u.s.w. in diesem Werk berechtigt auch ohne besondere Kennzeichnung nicht zu der Annahme, dass solche Namen im Sinne der Warenzeichen- und Markenschutzgesetzgebung als frei zu betrachten wären und daher von jedermann benutzt werden dürften.

Bibliographic information published by the Deutsche Nationalbibliothek: The Deutsche Nationalbibliothek lists this publication in the Deutsche Nationalbibliografie; detailed bibliographic data are available in the Internet at http://dnb.d-nb.de.

Any brand names and product names mentioned in this book are subject to trademark, brand or patent protection and are trademarks or registered trademarks of their respective holders. The use of brand names, product names, common names, trade names, product descriptions etc. even without a particular marking in this work is in no way to be construed to mean that such names may be regarded as unrestricted in respect of trademark and brand protection legislation and could thus be used by anyone.

Coverbild / Cover image: www.ingimage.com

Verlag / Publisher:
LAP LAMBERT Academic Publishing
ist ein Imprint der / is a trademark of
OmniScriptum GmbH & Co. KG
Bahnhofstraße 28, 66111 Saarbrücken, Deutschland / Germany
Email: info@lap-publishing.com

Herstellung: siehe letzte Seite /
Printed at: see last page
ISBN: 978-3-659-83025-9

Zugl. / Approved by: Tirana, University of Medical Tirana, 2015

ENIDA PETRO, PhD

EARLY CHILDHOOD CARIES
IN TIRANA, ALBANIA

MONOGRAPH

CONTENT

PREFACE.. 3
1. INTRODUCTION 4
2. PURPOSE OF STUDY.. 16
3. MATERIAL AND METHOD 17
4. RESULTS...26
5. DISCUSSION.. 51
6.CONCLUSION...60
7. RECOMMENDATIONS 61
8. REFERENCES 62
9. ANNEX 71

PREFACE

Early childhood caries, known in the literature as ECC (Early Childhood Caries) is a very serious problem in pediatric dentistry due to the rapid spreading of caries at an early age in the primary dentition. Children suffer the consequences of persistent pain and difficulties in feeding so they exhibit the phenomena of malnutrition and weight loss. ECC children have difficulty speaking and encounter social and psychological problems due to the distortion of the aesthetic appearance result of the dark-colored front teeth or their lack. Very often these children refuse to go to kindergarten or to socialize with their peers. In cases of complications as a result of not non-treatment of early childhood caries, local and general infections are very common and in exceptional cases they may also pose a risk to a child's life. Because of the children's young age, difficulties in managing them as well as lack of knowledge about this problem, many dentists recommend early removal of deciduous teeth causing irreversible damage to the permanent dentition.

In our daily practice of working with children very often we face such cases, but in the literature there are no data on the spread of the ECC to preschool aged children in our country. From information provided by some kindergartens in Tirana, it resulted that there is a continued lack of public service dental check-ups and teachers do not organize classes on oral health and hygiene. Also parents do not have complete information on the causes and consequences of ECC. This causes them to use wrong ways of nutrition and not properly care for the oral hygiene of their children. Parents are not aware of the age their child should visit the dentist for the first time and they know almost of no preventive measures which are available at that age such as fluoridation and silanation of deciduous teeth. As a result of this lack of knowledge and information children appear very late to the dentist and have to cope with uncomfortable curative procedures, especially at their age, which often cause refusal of treatment by the child. It was also noted that there was a lack of such information in the ranks of pediatricians, who on their part, must advise parents to consult a dentist in the very first year of a child's life. Also, it is important to pay attention to prenatal care as an one of the factors affecting the emergence of ECC from the first contact of the mother with the child right after birth. All this information should be part of preventive programs designed to improve the oral health of preschool children in our country.

1. INTRODUCTION

Early Childhood Caries, known in the literature as ECC is a destructive form of caries that affects the temporary teeth and may be present in children of very young age, and as early as teeth erupt (1, 2). The distinctive characteristic of caries in this age is that it affects initially a limited number of teeth which if not treated in time spread rapidly across all deciduous teeth (3).

1.1.   Definition of ECC

Early Childhood Caries is described in literature since 1952 from *Belteram* who used the term "les dent noire de tout-petits" which means "little children with black teeth" (4). The first proper definition of caries in young children was written in 1962 by *Fass*, who used the term "nursing bottle mouth" (5). Other definitions may be found in some terms used today such as "night bottle mouth", "nursing caries", "nursing bottle syndrome", "bottle mouth caries", "milk bottle syndrome", "baby bottle tooth decay" (6, 7). These definitions are used to identify the decay in children around the age of 5, who are bottle fed. In these cases, the teeth affected by caries are the maxillary incisive and molars. Mandibular incisors usually are not affected because of the position of the tongue during inhalation, protecting these teeth from the cariogenic effect of bottle contents (8, 9). In literature today we often encounter the term "rampant caries" (6, 9). This term is used to describe the more aggressive nature and the rapid progress within a short period of early childhood caries, from a single tooth in irreversible destruction of all deciduous teeth (Figure 1.1.1.).

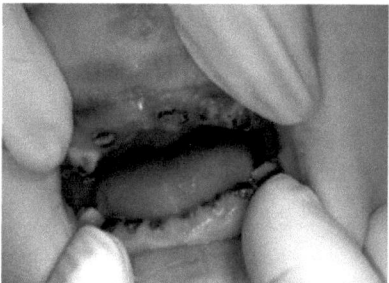

Figure 1.1.1. Clinical presentation of rampant caries.

In a workshop organized by the National Health Institute (NHI) in 1999 it was proposed that the term "Early Childhood Caries" – should be used to describe the presence of one or more decayed, filled or extracted primary teeth, because of the presence of caries in children as old as 71 months of age. (10)

According to the author *Gussy*, the presence of at least one carious lesion in the maxillary anterior in primary teeth in preschool children should be classified as ECC (11). The American Academy of Pediatric Dentistry (AAPD) defines ECC as the presence of at least one deciduous tooth affected by decay in children under 6 years of age (12).

1.2. ECC Classification

Different systems are used to classify early childhood caries (10, 13). The system most commonly used to classify ECC is the system determined in 2008 by AAPD (14). According to this classification we have:

Simple ECC - the presence of one or more cavitated, filled or removed teeth due to decay in children under 6 years; dmft <4 in children 3 years old, dmft <5 in children 4 years old or dmft <6 in children 5 years old.

Severe ECC – the presence of carious lesions as tender surfaces in children under 3 years; the presence of one or more maxillary anterior teeth that are cavitated, filled or removed due to caries in children 3 to 5 years; dmft ≥ 4 in children 3 years old, dmft ≥ 5 in children 4 years or dmft ≥ 6 in children 5 years old.

Maxillary ECC - the presence of one or more of the maxillary anterior teeth that are cavitated, filled or removed due to decay, in children under 6 years old.

1.3. Measuring ECC

The most common index used to measure dental caries in primary dentition the dmft / deft index. This index is based on the identification of dental caries in the past and in the present, including untreated caries prevalent in the present (dt) and caries treated in the past as we see teeth filled (ft) and teeth removed due to decay (mt/et). dmft /deft is the index used for years and is widely accepted throughout the world (15, 16). The diagnostic threshold recommended for epidemiological studies has been the dentine caries (17). The accuracy of enamel caries diagnosis is usually lower than that of the dentine caries (18). However there is evidence that a higher accuracy in establishing the diagnosis of enamel caries has been achieved through the proper training of the medical staff (19).

In order to estimate the ECC dissemination we measure its prevalence. Prevalence is the number of sick individuals in a population at a given point in time. Prevalence is usually reported as total number of sick cases per 1,000 subjects of the population and is expressed in percentage (20).

1.4. Global Prevalence of ECC

Dental caries has become a major public health concern, especially in developing countries, unlike developed countries where this problem is getting smaller and oral health is improving (21). Increasing urbanization and the rapid changes in food consumption are probably the factors that contribute to the deterioration of dental health in developing countries (22).

The prevalence of caries in developed countries is around 1-2%, while in developing countries and in some communities within the developed countries such as immigrants, minorities, etc., the prevalence increases up to 70% (23). While the literature has very few studies that determine the prevalence of ECC in children and the data usually refer to a wide age group such as the preschool children. These data show that overall prevalence of caries in preschool children has declined in most of developed countries (24, 25). While developing countries and in some cases even some developed countries, show a growing tendency (26, 27).

A detailed review of a large number of studies, with data on the ECC prevalence in Europe, Asia, Africa, the Middle East and North America showed that the highest prevalence of ECC was noticed in Africa and Southeast Asia (28). The results of studies conducted in several European countries such as England, Sweden and Finland have shown that the prevalence of ECC in 3 year old children, ranges from 1% to 32% (23, 29, 30), while in Eastern Europe ECC prevalence is 56% (31). In the United States the prevalence of caries in preschool children is 17%, though some studies show that the prevalence of ECC varies from 4% to 90% in some communities of Native American population (7, 29, 32, 33, 34). In Latin America the prevalence of ECC was 46% in children 25-36 months (35), while in Canada in 3 year old children the prevalence of ECC was 67% (36).

Studies conducted in Asian countries show that the prevalence of ECC in 3 year old children is highest in the region of the Far East and it ranges from 36% to 85% (30, 37, 38, 39, 40, 41) while in India the prevalence of ECC in children 8-48 months is 44% (42). In the Middle East ECC prevalence in 3 year old children varies from 22% to 61% (43, 44, 45) and in Africa from 38% to 45% (46, 46). Conclusions based on the results of these studies show that early childhood caries is considered an epidemic in developing countries (48).

1.5.   ECC Prevalence in Albania

Our literature offers no data regarding the prevalence of early childhood caries in preschool age groups in children 3-5 years. This is the most important age to assess the level of presence and development of ECC because primary dentition is fully formed and the first permanent molar tooth has not yet erupted.

A single study has been conducted in children 1-3 years old in kindergartens in Tirana in 2010 and it found that the presence of ECC has been observed in 47% of children participating in the study (49).

1.6.   ECC Etiology

Early childhood caries has a multifactorial etiology where several key and determining factors are involved such as: dental structure, carbohydrates enzyme, microorganisms and time. Also in the emergence and development of ECC several other factors have a significant impact, being those risky or helpful factors such as age, sex, race or ethnicity, genetics, socio-economic status and behavior (7).

1.6.1. Dental Structure

Early childhood caries may appear immediately after the teeth have erupted. The surface of the teeth emerged is not yet fully matured and this is the main reason that these teeth are easily affected by caries (9). Once the tooth has fully emerged, the enamel surface undergoes the final stages of post-eruptive maturation and final mineralization stage. It is precisely during this intermediate period, following the release of the tooth and before final maturity time, when deciduous teeth are more sensitive and may easily be affected by early childhood caries. The presence of defects in the structure of enamel formation increases the risk of ECC. Traumas and infections associated with them are also responsible for many of localized defects in the dental structure (50).

However the main cause of proliferation early childhood caries is the presence of Streptococcus Mutans and carbohydrate enzyme (21). Oral level of this bacterium, which is usually transmitted from the mother, has proved to be higher in children affected by ECC (51). Irregular surfaces as spots, fissures and pits that are highly expressed in deciduous teeth serve as places for retention of plaque bringing increased levels of Streptococcus Mutans and the reduction or elimination of carbohydrates enzyme.

1.6.1. Carbohydrates enzyme

Early childhood caries is closely related to carbohydrates that are active in the daily diet. Microorganisms found in the oral cavity, particularly Streptococcus mutans, use these carbohydrates to form an adhesive layer that allows them to adhere to the tooth surface. From the process of fermentation of carbohydrates organic acids are produced, which initially demineralize the dental enamel (52). Continuous consumption of carbohydrates in liquid form is a high risk factor that affects the appearance of the ECC due to prolonged contact with the surface of the tooth (53).

Maxillary anterior caries prevalence is higher in children who use the bottle of milk sweetened or with other sugary drinks than in children who use a bottle of milk without added sugar or simply with water (7). The frequency of sucrose intake is actually more important than the total amount consumed (11). Results of a study conducted in Jordan in 2005 indicated that a higher prevalence of ECC was observed in children with higher consumption of enwrapped sweets (54). Also the use of a "soothing" pacifier coated with sugar or honey which was given to young children to calm their crying or before sleep is a risk factor for the emergence of ECC (53).

Sanctions imposed by the United Nations (UN), to reduce sugary products, facilitated a decrease in cases of caries in Iraqi children for a period of over 5 years (55).

Although breast milk is very important to ensure the best nutrition for infants, frequent breast feeding during the day and especially at night when the baby teeth have emerged, may affect the appearance of ECC. Breast milk contains twice the amount of lactose than the milk of cattle and causes a greater reduction of pH in the plaque and thus will result in a greater demineralization or decalcification of dental enamel (56).

Fruit juices and sugary drinks play a significant role in the emergence of early childhood caries. Natural fruit juices contain fructose which has a high acidic action. While in sugary beverages a sweetening agent usually sucrose is added which in turn enhances the acidic action even more. Fruit juices and sugary drinks cause a significant decrease in pH of the plaque (21). When these are consumed by children who show the first signs of ECC, enamel erosion ECC progresses rapidly and spreads its most aggressive form known as "rampant caries" (9).

1.6.3. Microorganisms

Microorganisms responsible for dental caries can be transmitted from person to person. This transmission in the cases of early childhood caries is usually from mother to child through saliva (8). This is called vertical transmission and can occur through kissing mouth to mouth especially when the child puts his fingers in his mouth after he had them in the mouth of the mother or when the mother cleans the bottle with her saliva (57).

Many studies have shown that children carry a huge amount of Streptococcus Mutans in the oral cavity, which is capable of producing a high level of acid, mainly lactic acid, causing temporary tooth demineralization (58). Today it is believed that Streptococcus Mutans adherence to bacterial plaque is independent of the presence of sucrose and is directly mediated by salivary proteins, which form the pellicle on the surface of the tooth. The amount of Streptococcus Mutans increases with age and with the increase in the number of teeth emerged. The earlier the colonization of these microorganisms in the oral cavity of the child occurs, the higher is the risk for the emergence of ECC. For this reason today's early childhood caries is considered a transmitted infectious disease, where the Streptococcus Mutans is the main responsible bacterium for the infection (59).

A study conducted in Tirana highlighted the role of Streptococcus Mutans as the main cause of early childhood caries. In this study the presence and the average level of Streptococcus Mutans in saliva was recorded in the majority of children with ECC and also for their mothers. The results showed a significant correlation between Streptococcus Mutans vertical transmission from mother to child and early childhood caries. Results were confirmed not only clinically but also statistically and they indicated that high level of Streptococcus Mutans is associated with the high risk of ECC occurrence (60).

Another way of transmission of Streptococcus Mutans is the horizontal transmission from child to child within the same family, between siblings or within of the same social group as in the case of children attending nurseries and kindergartens, but this way of transmission is not amply proved and literature does not provide clear evidence on this matter (59).

1.6.4. Time

Time is an important factor in the development of ECC associated with the frequency and amount of the sugary juice consumed daily. Data from the survey showed that children with ECC in average use the bottlefed or breastfed 8.3 times a day, while children with no signs of ECC use it only 2.2 times a day (8). The frequency of contact of deciduous teeth with sugary products within 24 hours has a significant impact on the development of early childhood caries. When the quantity of milk or sugary liquids consumed by children is divided into smaller portions there is a greater decrease of pH of the plaque than when the same amount is consumed all at once (8).

Timing is also a very important factor while bottle-feeding or breast-feeding or during the absorption of the sugar coated "soothing" pacifier by the child, which affects both the extent of the lesion as well as the number of teeth affected by early childhood caries. An important aspect to be considered during bottle-feeding is the longevity of the constant contact of the bottle with teeth, especially during sleep. Constant suction of the bottle content throughout the night directly affects the appearance of ECC (7).

Also the use of prolonged breast-feeding after the age of one and also breast-feeding the child at night after the age of 6 months is ranked in the literature as a high risk factor for the emergence of early childhood caries (61). The presence of ECC in breastfed children is caused not only because the mother is available throughout the day, whenever the baby asks to be fed, but also because she uses breastfeeding throughout the night to put the child to sleep, or to calm the crying baby (61).

A study conducted in Tirana highlighted a moderate link between ECC and breastfeeding after age one year old, but this relationship proved significant in the case of prolonged breast-feeding which occurred at different times of day and night, whenever the child needed soothing (62).

1.6.5. Age

Early childhood caries affects the primary dental system in children under 6 years and may appear as soon as teeth erupt (1, 2, 12). The surface of the teeth emerged is not fully matured and this is the main reason that these teeth are easily affected by ECC (9). Irregular surfaces such as spots, fissures and cavities which are very pronounced in deciduous teeth serve as retention areas of the bacterial plaque. Carbohydrate consumption is greater during early childhood and proper oral hygiene is achieved with more difficulty. According to the AAPD the age group of 2-3 years, encounters the highest risk for early childhood caries (12).

1.6.6. Gender

There is no clear evidence we can use to determine any significant differences in early childhood, among males and females in terms of the prevalence of ECC. Slightly higher values of the prevalence of ECC in females are believed to be the result of earlier eruption of deciduous teeth in females.

1.6.7. Race and ethnicity

The influence of race and ethnicity in the prevalence of ECC deals with cultural influences and different lifestyles (7). The literature provides evidence that minorities face an increased risk for early childhood caries (63, 64). However, in a study conducted in 2003, by *Montero*, he found no significant difference in the level of ECC when he considered ethnicity as a factor (65). While in migrant population, there is a significant link with a higher prevalence of early childhood caries (66). According to some authors it is difficult to determine the impact of race and ethnicity in the prevalence of ECC due to the incorrect definition of ethnicity. In several cases the sample population participant in the study was grouped by nationality and in other cases by origin. Also, according to several authors what makes this variable more difficult to determine is the impact of confounding factors such as the nutrition habits and oral hygiene (67). Often these minorities are the most discriminated strata and have the lowest socio- economic status that impacts the greater prevalence of early childhood caries (68).

1.6.8. Genetics

Genetic factors are believed to influence the prevalence of early childhood caries through inherited or acquired immune system resistance and dental structure, the morphology of the surface of the tooth or their placement in the arcade (69).

1.6.9. Socio-economic status

Socio-economic status (SES) shows the level of education, level of income and employment of a single individual or group of individuals (70, 71). Individuals with low SES have social and financial disadvantages that reduce their ability to take care of themselves, get professional quality service and live in a healthy environment. These individuals are likely to neglect oral health problems, the need for care and prevention for themselves and their children. Low level of education also increases the prevalence of dental caries (72, 73). Low SES increases the level of risk for ECC (7, 74). This effect is caused by the difference in nutrition habits and the role of carbohydrates in people's diet (18). Experiencing caries and the frequency of consumption of sugar is higher in children of parents with lower educational level (75). According to some authors, disparities in oral health result from the use of milk with added sugar and lack of fluorinated toothpaste (76).

Early childhood caries is most prevalent among children born to single mothers, who live in poverty or in poor economic conditions or whose parents have low levels of education, especially among the uneducated and illiterate mothers (77). Mother's care directly affects the child's oral health and level of dmft (78). Mothers with low levels of education tend to give their children sugary products or packaged foods between meals, while mothers with higher education level prefer home food or fresh fruit (79).

Malnourished children during the pre, peri or post natal period and those with lower weight birth run a higher risk of having teeth with deficient mineralization, which are more easily affected by colonization of Streptococcus Mutans and early childhood caries (80).

1.6.10. Behavior

The presence of dental caries displayed in the early childhood is closely related to behavior patterns (73, 81). The main factors associated with behavior are feeding habits, diet, amount of sugar consumed, dental plaque control, optimal exposure to fluoride and oral health care (82).

A pattern in the model of behavior has to do with lifestyle. The literature emphasizes the importance of family influence in the development of a model of proper and healthy behavior since early childhood (83, 84). Since the most dominating environment in the child's life is family, family members, especially mothers have a direct impact on a child's learning and motivation habits of oral health care. Parents transmit to their children the same customs they themselves observe in everyday life due to the influence of the surrounding environment, culture or their personal beliefs (85). Mothers who carry out regular periodic check-ups to the dentist are more likely to see a dentist for their child's first visit and are more interested in continuing to seek professional care (86, 87). A study conducted in Tirana in 2009, showed that only 12% of parents had taken their child for the first visit to the dental cabinet no later than age 1 year. Also this study showed that the average age of the first visit of children was 7 years and the main reason for this delay in 98% of cases, was the fear that the parents themselves had experienced from the first meeting with the dentist (88).

Nutrition habits of infant and the use of sugary foods and drinks in early childhood are closely linked to the beliefs and practices handed down over the generations from mothers to daughters (89, 90). In several surveys conducted during the preparation of this doctoral thesis, the significant impact of nutrition and dietary habits in the prevalence of early childhood caries was observed (91, 92, 93, 94).

1.7. ECC Clinic

Initially opaque white spots appear only in the upper centrals incisors. Later these spots become a dark brown color and around this same time early childhood caries stars affecting respectively the occlusal surfaces of the upper molars, the canine vestibular sites and the lower molar. Very soon all the surfaces of deciduous teeth are affected and ECC spreads deeper without causing any significant symptoms (95). Dental crowns of deciduous teeth are completely destroyed (Figure 1.7.1.). Later pulpo - periodontal infections appear which are often accompanied by pain, swelling and fistulas. Untreated cases often lead to abscess complications and phlegmon affecting the general condition of the child.

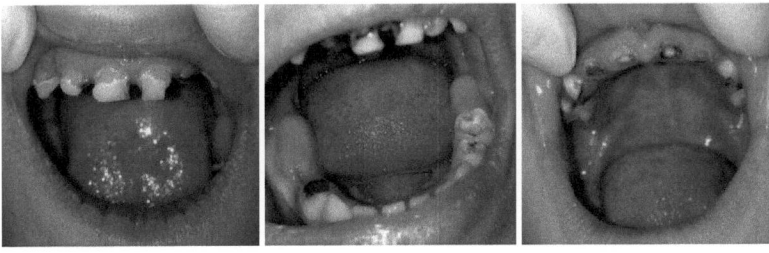

Figure 1.7.1. Clinical presentation of ECC.

1.8. ECC Identification

Identification of ECC in the early stages is a prerequisite for success in the treatment and prevention of further spread of ECC. Therefore the child's first visit to the dental cabinet is very important. It is recommended that the first dental visit should be as soon as the child's first tooth comes out and no later than the age of 1 year (96, 97, 98). The literature suggests that early childhood caries should be classified as a pediatric problem in addition to it being a dental problem and pediatricians should play an important role in identifying the ECC, as pediatric doctors are the ones more frequently in contact with children and their parents (99, 100).

1.9. ECC Treatment

Treatment of early childhood caries is multi-factorial and involves the child, his parents and the specialized dental personnel to ensure that restorative treatment will be supported by prevention, oral hygiene and proper nutritional habits (101.102).

In initial carious lesions minimal restorative intervention techniques such as ART techniques are applied in order to reduce trauma to the child and the parent (80). This technique is accomplished by placing glass ionomer cement into the cavity without the use of the cutter or the local anesthetic (103). In other cases where the lesion has progresses deeper the recommended treatment is the technique of coverage with a paste containing steroid antibiotics such as Ledermix or Septomixine Forte pastes. In cases when the carious cavity is open the method recommended is the initial cleaning with an excavator, antibiotic paste placement and temporary closure with glass ionomer cement. This method favors the reduction of Streptococcus mutans in the cavity, reducing tooth sensitivity and serves as desensitization method for the child. Later it comes the final filling with restorative materials or stainless steel crowns according to relevant procedures (95). While in advanced stages, when the ECC complications appear, it is necessary to apply endodontic techniques under local anesthetic effects (104). A study conducted in Tirana showed that the use of these pastes containing steroid antibiotics is the most effective method in the treatment of ECC complications (105).

When the child cooperation is difficult due to the young age of the child, his agitated stage or when we are treating cases of children with mental disabilities, the recommended method of treatment is sedation or general anesthesia. Many of these treatments are impossible for some children in developing countries due to the high financial costs or lack of specialized dental staff (106).

1.10. ECC Consequences

In most cases children suffering from ECC are not treated in a timely or proper manner due to lack of information of parents, the young age of children, difficulties in management, and lack of specialized professional service as well as the high cost of service. Because of the difficult experiences and the need for frequent visits to the dental cabinet, the child refuses treatment or leaves in the middle of treatment procedures which lead to disappointment or to the disruption child – dentist relationship. This often results in premature deciduous teeth extractions as shown in Figure 1.10.1.

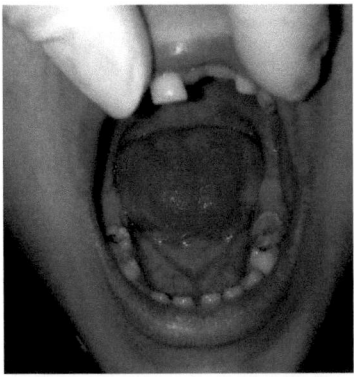

Figura 1.10.1. Premature extraction of tooth 61.

These cases are mostly associated with abnormalities of the chronology such as premature eruptions or delays in the emergence of permanent teeth. Also the risk of the appearance of carious lesions in the first permanent molar is much higher among children with ECC. In our clinical experience with these children we have identified many cases with the presence of dental caries in occlusal surfaces of permanent molars, just erupted (Figure 1.10.2.).

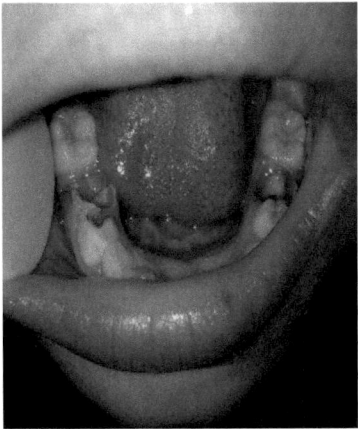

Figure 1.10.2. The presence of caries in first permanent molars.

1.11. ECC Prevention

Preventive strategies are divided into two main groups: strategies that apply to the population of all individuals affected or not by the disease and risk strategies that are directed only toward at-risk groups or individuals (98, 107). Population strategies include fluoridation of drinking water, the use of fluorinated toothpaste and oral health education (98, 108). While risk strategies seek to protect individuals who may be affected by caries due to the transformation of risk factors (107). The effectiveness of risk strategies is being questioned in many studies and the accuracy of defining individuals or at- risk groups is low (109).

The main methods for prevention of ECC usually focus on reducing the use of carbohydrates, reducing the microbial load, increasing tooth resistance or a combination of them (89, 110). These methods include methods addressing the community, professional clinical methods and methods of personal home care (98, 111).

Methods addressed to the community are usually applied by public health authorities and other government bodies at the national level such as those dealing with educational programs and fluoridation of drinking water. Professional methods are applied in dental clinics by the medical personnel and they deal with topical fluoridation and placement of dental sealants in the temporary dental system, while at home are applied preventive methods relating to personal care of oral hygiene, nutrition and dietary habits.

Educational programs consist of information summaries conducted through conversations, learning activities, exchange of experiences and they focus mainly on changing the child nutritional habits and reducing the level of Streptococcus mutans (51, 112). These programs aim to provide advice on reducing the frequency of daily intake of sugary beverages and foods, daily brushing of teeth with fluorinated toothpastes and regular visits to the dentist (113, 114).

Prevention of ECC is made possible through education of young parents and prospective parents on methods of nutrition, abstinence from cariogenic foods, oral hygiene and the use of fluoride in their children (115, 116, 117, 118, 119) .

Fluoridation of drinking water is a systemic prevention method involving the whole community, but in recent decades this method has lower efficiency in reducing the ECC due to scarce natural resources of fluorinated water and replacement of fluoride intake through other means such as those with local effect (98, 109, 111, 120, 121).

Local methods of prevention include the fluorinated toothpaste, mouth rinse aid, fluorinated gels and varnishes. Usage of fluorinated toothpaste seems to be the local method with the lowest cost and highest efficiency in the prevention of ECC, therefore, it is the most common method and can be widely used by all children (89, 120, 122, 123, 124). Fluorinated rinses also have daily or weekly use and help in the prevention of ECC and they are usually free in many countries that apply this method in preschool children, but it may easily be applied at home under the care of parents or guardians of the child (125). The effectiveness of these methods of self-care at home, which relate to the oral hygiene for young children, depends on the care and knowledge of parents and guardians involved in raising the child, and can be improved under the influence of educational advisory and training programs (110, 126, 127, 128, 129).

Methods of professional clinical care deal with the application of fluorinated gels and varnishes in preschool children. These methods should be applied especially in those children who encounter e higher risk for early childhood caries. In developed countries these methods are widely are applied and free of charge by dental hygienists who perform periodical check-ups in children of preschool age (69).

Applying sealants in primary dental system is also another very important method of used in professional dental care. According to the AAPD and ADA, retention of sealants in deciduous teeth it is higher than in permanent teeth because at the time of sealant application deciduous teeth have fully erupted and their crown is fully formed (96, 97, 130). Different studies show that 68% of the deciduous teeth with sealant application are not affected by ECC (131). A study conducted by Tirana is noted the efficiency of sealant application in the prevention of ECC (132).

2. PURPOSE OF STUDY

2.1. General Purpose

The purpose of this study is to determine the prevalence and severity of early childhood caries in children 3-5 years old in the public kindergartens in Tirana.

2.2. Specific Objectives

Specific objectives of this study are:

1. To determine the distribution of ECC according to AAPD methods used for classification in the study subjects.

2. To determine the dental status and carious experience in deciduous teeth in children 3-5 years old in the public kindergartens in Tirana.

3. To set the deft index and Care Index (CI).

4. To determine the risk factors for early childhood caries.

5. To determine the distribution of study subjects according to these factors.

6. To evaluate the association between these factors and early childhood caries.

7. To evaluate the association between these factors and deft index.

8. To assess the association between these factors and the level of care.

9. To analyze and compare the results with the well-known literature references.

10. To draw the necessary conclusions based on the data results.

11. To recommend prevention strategies that aid in the prevention of early childhood caries.

3. MATERIALS AND METHODS

3.1. Type of study

This is a transversal epidemiological study type (cross - sectional). The superiority of this type of study consists in the acquisition of point information (at a certain point in time) about the size (magnitude) or the prevalence of a particular characteristic or specific health event in the population of interest. It is this feature of transversal studies in this paper which was used to assess the prevalence of early childhood caries in children aged 3-5 years in the city of Tirana.

3.2. Period of study

The entire study duration was about 3 years. It began in September 2011 and was completed in late 2014. The intraoral examination process and registration of children in selected kindergartens lasted for a period of 3 months.

3.3. Characteristics of the sample population

This study was conducted in Tirana, Albania's capital (Figure 3.3.1.). About 30% of the population lives in Tirana.

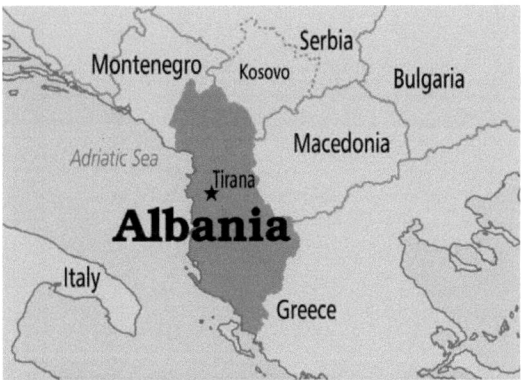

Figure 3.3.1. The map of Tirana (Albania).

The study was conducted only in public kindergartens. Private kindergartens were not included in this study because there is no accurate data or a complete list of private kindergartens and the exact number of children enrolled. Also, we considered the fact that not all kindergartens are registered and licensed. In any case, the generalization of the results of this study will refer to public kindergartens in the city of Tirana. From this point of view, the exclusion of private kindergartens from this study is no threat to the validity of the paper as a whole. According to information received in the Regional Education Directorate in Tirana, the city has 42 public kindergartens with 7232 children enrolled. That list served as the sampling frame in the current study.

This study included children 3-5 years because at this age group all deciduous teeth have erupted and it is the appropriate age for their study according to WHO criteria (17). In this age group we may asses the spread of early childhood caries based on the ECC classification as defined in 2008 by the AAPD (14).

3.4. Selection of the study sample

According to the list provided by the Regional Education Directorate in Tirana, out of 42 kindergartens 4 were randomly selected according by using the "probability proportionate to size" (probability proportional to size) method in our selection. Kindergarten s selected were those with no. 11, 18, 31 and 35. These represent some of the very best kindergartens Tirana.

During our preliminary visits to these kindergartens we found out that Kindergarten no.18 was "hosting" Kindergarten no.40 due to reconstruction of the latter. Also, Kindergarten no.22 was "hosting" the Kindergarten no.35 for the same reason. Both "guest" kindergartens were included in the study.

Kindergarten Directorates provided information on the number of children enrolled, the number of children actively attending and the number of children who only attended daily. These data are presented in Table 3.4.1.

Table 3.4.1. Number of children in kindergartens included in the study.

Kindergarten no.	Address	Registered	Active attendees (approximatly)	Daily attendees (approximatly)
11	"K. e Parisit"	232	220	200
18	"M. Grameno"	243	230	200
22	"K. Manastirit"	208	190	170
31	"P. Bogdani"	275	245	235
35	"guest" to 22	169	160	150
40	"guest" to 18	96	80	65
Total		1223	1125	1020

3.5. The sample size in this study

The sample size was estimated by WIN program - PEPI (133). According to sample size calculations done a priori and based on conservative assumptions, the minimum sample size for this survey was 734. Conservative assumptions tend to maximize sample size. In this regard, a size of 734 children was estimated as the maximum possible to achieve the purpose and objectives of this study. However, it was decided to include a number of 1000 children in order to increase the power of the study and also was taken into account the refusal rate, the absence of children in the kindergartens on the day of the examination and the possibility of exclusion of children who did not submit their questionnaire completed by parents.

In total the study included 904 children, who were present in the respective kindergartens on the day of examination, children who did not refuse the examination and had submitted the questionnaire completed by parents. So, the participation rate in the study was 90.4% and the final sample of this study (n = 904) was of a much larger size than the minimum required (n = 734) to achieve the purpose and objectives of this study.

3.6. Data collection

The collection of the necessary information for this study was conducted with the approval of the Regional Education Directorate in Tirana and the relevant departments of kindergartens selected for this study. The collection of these data was conducted through structured questionnaires completed by parents and children's intraoral examination in each kindergarten.

3.6.1. Questionnaires used in the study

A questionnaire was prepared for the purposes of this study. It was structured in line with certain models used in similar studies (72, 134, 135, 136, and 137). The questionnaire is included in the annex section at the end of the paper. The questionnaire contained inquiries about general information such as the name of the child and the mother / guardian and phone number. The questions were short and often required only the alternative yes or no answer. Responses were to be completed by the parent / guardian of the child in the box blank and mark it with X, or in writing in the case of explanatory answers. The survey questions were clear and easy to understand and interpret on the part of parents and intended to collect information on some important data such as socio-economic status of the mother / guardian, the child's health, feeding habits, oral hygiene and oral health care.

Questionnaires prepared (n = 1300) were submitted to the relevant departments of each kindergarten according to the number of children enrolled. The total number of questionnaires was bigger than the total number of children enrolled to provide for any any potential loss or damage during its administration, distribution or return. Administered questionnaires were distributed and reconvened from educators. Despite numerous efforts and difficulties encountered the majority of parents (n = 978) completed and submitted the questionnaires.

3.6.2. Examination methods used in the study

This study used the intraoral examination of all kindergarten children selected as the method for diagnosing early childhood caries. Registration and examination was carried out by two screeners, who had been informed in advance of the criteria for registration, screening and diagnosis based on the WHO (17) standards, and were familiar with the methods and means that would be used during the registration and examination. Calibration of screeners was conducted through a test session which was held for the registration and examination of a limited number of children (n = 20) divided equally for each doctor. This session was conducted in the third group of Kindergarten no.31 before the start of the process.

The process of registration and intraoral examination and took a few days for each of the selected kindergartens and lasted for a period of 3 months. The process of examination included only children (n = 923) who were present on the day of the examination and had submitted a questionnaire completed by parents. Initially the children were given a short presentation in the form of conversation about oral health and dental care (Figure 3.6.2.1.).

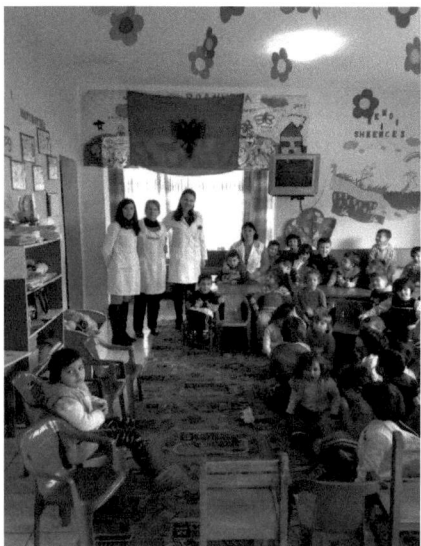

Figure 3.6.2.1. Communicating with children before exmination

The examination procedure was initially tested in children who were not afraid and wanted to be included in the examination. In such cases the examination was conducted in a playful mode, without wearing a mask or an apron (Figure 3.6.2.2.). However in some cases (n = 19) children refused to be examined, especially in the younger groups because of fear from the procedure.

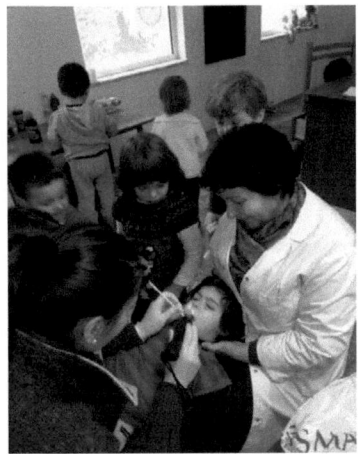

Figure 3.6.2.2. Testing the examination procedure in children.

During the examination the children sat in the chair opposite the examiner using the method knee-to-knee position (Figure 3.6.2.3.). In the case of younger children lap-to-lap position method was used, where the child is in a position lying in the lap of a teacher who sits in the chair opposite from the examiner (Figure 3.6.2.4.).

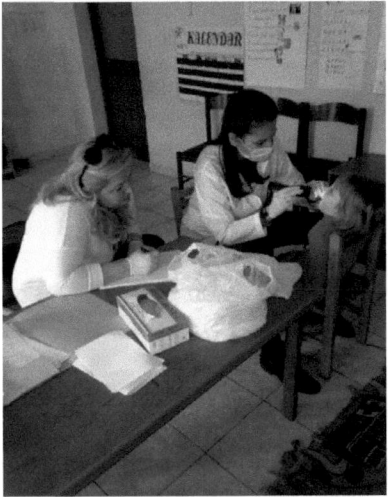

Figure 3.6.2.3. Using the knee-to-knee position.

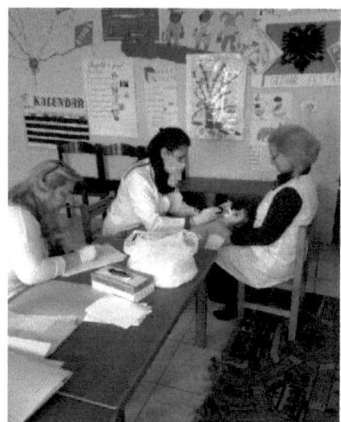

Figure 3.6.2.4. Using the lap-to-lap position.

During intraoral examination dentists wore mask, gloves and used disposable plastic instruments. The instruments were packaged in a kit containing the mirror, probe and forceps (Figure 3.6.2.5.). Initially the teeth were kept dry with cotton pads or rolls. A LED flashlight was used as the light source, focusing on the oral cavity. All tools were placed on top of a desk (Figure 3.6.2.6.). Diagnosis of early childhood caries was carried through the examination of deciduous teeth by using a mirror and probe.

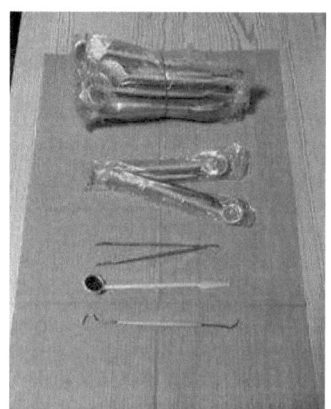

Figure 3.6.2.5. Disposable plastic instruments
(Shenzhen YouYou Co., LTD).

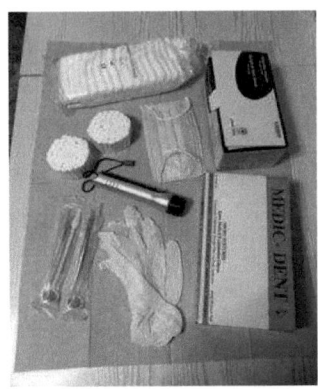

Figure 3.6.2.6. Tools used in the intraoral examination.

The data for each child were recorded in the file type compiled beforehand. This dental file is presented in the annex section at the end of this paper. Each card had a serial number in order to identify each child. In the top part of the card was marked the date, the number of kindergarten, child's name and surname, age and gender. According to WHO criteria age is recorded based on the child's last birthday (17). In our case children who turned 3 were marked with the number 3, children who had turned 4 were marked with the number 4, and 5 for children who had turned 5 years based on census data for each child. The second part of the card marked the dental status presented in a scheme with empty boxes for each temporary tooth marked with numbers by the FDI counting system. The examination included only the teeth of the primary dental system and their condition was marked with codes following WHO criteria (17). ECC form was marked for each child based on the classification criteria set out in 2008 by the AAPD (18).

After the examination procedure was concluded the total number of children (n = 904) who were examined was estimated, and the data was recorded in the relevant files. This was the final number of children involved in the study. Comprehensive data in absolute figures are presented in Table 3.6.2.1.

Table 3.6.2.1. Summary data on the study subjects.

Total number of children registered in kindergartens	1223
Total number of questionnaires submitted to kindergartens	1300
Total number of questionnaires filled by parents	978
Total number of children examined (children who were present and had filled questionnaires)	923
Total number of children who refused examination	19
Total number of children registered and examined (children included in the study)	904

Figure 3.6.2.7. presents some of the cases of ECC found in children during the examination procedure.

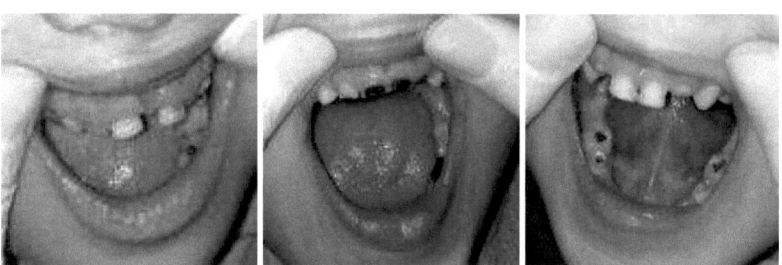

Figure 3.6.2.7. Presence of ECC in children examined.

3.6.3. Examination credibility

To assess the credibility of the examination, 5% -10% of subjects in the study, but not less than 25 entities would undergo a double screening (17). In our study some of the children (n = 96) in each kindergarten, were re-examined by a second examiner and the data was re-registered in another folder. The data were collected in order to help calculate the Kappa index for comparing deft index values based on the interpretation by Landis and Koch (138). These data are presented in Table 3.6.3.1.

Table 3.6.3.1. KAPPA Index interpretation according to Landis and Koch

KAPPA Index value	Interpretation
≤ 0	Lack of compatibility
0.01 – 0.20	Very low compatibility
0.21 – 0.40	Low compatibility
0.41 – 0.60	Moderate compatibility
0.61 – 0.80	High compatibility
0.81 – 1.00	Absolute compatibility

3.7. Selection of variables for the study

Variables that were included in the study were chosen in such a way as to contribute in achieving the objectives of the study to evaluate the link (association) between the disease as the dependent variable and the disease exposure factors which are independent variables (139). In this study we will analyze the relationship between early childhood caries (the dependent variable) and risk factors such as demographic, socio – economic factors, as well as those related to the medical history, eating habits, oral hygiene and oral health care (independent variables).

3.8. Statistical analysis of the data in the study

Statistical analysis was conducted in SPSS (Statistical Package for the Social Sciences, version 15.0). Size of central tendency was calculated for numerical variables (arithmetic average, median and the mode) and also the dispersion size (variance, standard deviation and interquartile distance). Absolute values and their respective percentages were calculated for categorical variables. Comparison of the average values between the two groups was made possible through the test "t" test of Student and Mann - Whitney (a non-parametric version of the test "t" Student). Comparison of proportions (percentages) for categorical variables was made possible through Hi square test and Fisher's exact test. The general linear model was used to calculate the average values of the indexes. Average values and respective confidence interval 95% were calculated for all indicators. In all cases, it was considered statistically significant a value of $p \leq 0:05$. The results were presented in absolute values and in percentage and illustrated by tables.

4. RESULTS

4.1. Assessment of the examination credibility

The coefficient of compatibility beyond chance (Kappa Index) between the two experts involved in the study is presented in Table 4.1.1. As may be seen from the table, this coefficient ranges from 0699 to date until 0802 index of deft index. These results represent a moderate to high compatibility, which means that the examination is reliable.

Table 4.1.1. KAPPA Index (compatibility beyond chance)

Variable	KAPPA Index
deft index	0.802
ft index	0.701
et index	0.766
dt index	0.699

4.2. The prevalence of Early Childhood Caries (ECC)

Table 4.2.1. presents early childhood caries (ECC) in the children involved in the study, the absolute number, average value, standard deviation and minimum and maximum value.

Table 4.2.1. Early Childhood Caries in the study subjects.

Number	904
Average	2.7
Standard deviation	0.749
Minimum	1
Maximum	4

By analyzing the collected data we were able to report the overall prevalence of early childhood caries in children included in this study.

The prevalence of Early Childhood Caries (ECC)
in 3 - 5 year old children in Tirana public kindergartens:
823/904 = 91%

Table 4.2.2. presents in detail in absolute numbers and relevant percentages, the distribution of early childhood caries according to the ECC classification defined in 2008 by the AAPD (18). The table shows that most of the children involved in this study (62.1%) suffer from a severe form of the ECC.

Table 4.2.2. Distribution of ECC in the study subjects based on the AADP classification.

Variable	Number	Percentage (%)
ECC Form:		
Without ECC	81	9.0
Simple ECC	184	20.4
Severe ECC	561	62.1
Maxillary ECC	78	8.6

4.3. deft index

By analyzing the data collected we were able to report average values 6.2, 0.07 and 0.2 respectively for specific indexes dt, et and ft, and the average value 6.45 of the deft index. Table 4.3.1. presents the average values for dt, t, ft and deft indexes, and the standard deviation for each index, while Table 4.3.2. shows the distribution date, t, ft and deft indexes in children involved in the study.

Table 4.3.1. Average value of dt, et, ft and deft index.

	dt index	et index	ft index	deft index
Number	904	904	904	904
Average	6.20	0.07	0.20	6.45
Standard deviation	4.236	0.424	0.781	4.258

Table 4.3.2. Distribution of dt, et, ft and deft index in children included in the study.

Value	Index			
	dt	et	ft	deft
0	87 (9.5)*	867 (95.8)	826 (91.4)	80 (8.8)
1	26 (2.9)	23 (2.5)	32 (3.5)	24 (2.7)
2	102 (11.3)	11 (1.2)	19 (2.1)	92 (10.2)
3	36 (4.0)	2 (0.2)	11 (1.2)	37 (4.1)
4	116 (12.8)	-	8 (0.9)	105 (11.6)
5	47 (5.2)	-	6 (0.7)	49 (5.4)
6	95 (10.5)	-	1 (0.1)	99 (11.0)
7	46 (5.1)	-	-	38 (4.2)
8	113 (12.5)	-	1 (0.1)	125 (13.6)
9	37 (4.1)	1 (0.1)	-	38 (4.2)
10	73 (8.1)	-	-	78 (8.6)
11	17 (1.9)	-	-	15 (1.7)
12	52 (5.8)	-	-	62 (6.9)
13	8 (0.9)	-	-	10 (1.1)
14	24 (2.7)	-	-	28 (3.1)
15	1 (0.1)	-	-	1 (0.1)
16	8 (0.9)	-	-	7 (0.8)
17	1 (0.1)	-	-	-
18	3 (0.3)	-	-	3 (0.3)
19	-	-	-	-
20	12 (1.3)	-	-	13 (1.4)
Total	904 (100)	904 (100)	904 (100)	904 (100)

* The absolute value and percentage (in parentheses)

4.4. Care Index CI

Table 4.4.1. presents the CI index value in absolute numbers and average value, together with deviation or standard deviation and also the minimum and maximum values. These data show that the average value of Care Index is 3.1%, meaning only 3.1% of the affected deciduous teeth are treated.

Table 4.4.1. Value of CI (Care Index).

Number	904
Average	3.1
Standard deviation	3.52

4.5. Demographic characteristics of the study subjects

4.5.1. The distribution of subjects by demographic characteristics

Table 4.5.1.1. presents the demographic characteristics of the children included in our study. The data collected shows that about 20% of the children were 3 years old, 34% were 4 years old and 46% were 5 years old. With regard to gender distribution, we may say that the male / female representation balance was almost complete.

Table 4.5.1.1. Distribution of study subjects by demographic characteristics and respective preschool educational institution.

Variable	Number	Percentage
Age:		
3 years	178	19.7
4 years	308	34.1
5 years	418	46.2
Gender:		
Male	454	50.2
Female	450	49.8
Kindergarten No.:		
11	185	20.5
18	157	17.4
22	160	17.7
31	201	22.2
35	140	15.5
40	61	6.7

4.5.2. Distribution of ECC by demographic characteristics

Table 4.5.2.1. presents ECC distribution in the subjects involved in the study by age, which shows a significant statistical association with the increase in the age of the child, ECC is more pronounced.

Table 4.5.2.1. ECC Distribution based on the age of study subjects.

Variable	No ECC	Simple ECC	Severe ECC	Maxillary ECC	p - value
3 years	26 (32.1)	26 (14.1)	102 (18.2)	24 (30.8)*	
4 years	40 (49.4)	67 (36.4)	175 (31.2)	26 (33.3)	p<0.001§
5 years	15 (18.5)	91 (49.5)	284 (50.6)	28 (35.9)	

§ The value of p according to Hi square test.
* Absolute numbers and percentages in parentheses.

Table 4.5.2.2. presents ECC distribution of children participating in the study by gender, which showed no statistical association, meaning that both males and females are affected in the same extent by early childhood caries.

Table 4.5.2.2. ECC Distribution according to gender of study subjects.

Variable	No ECC	Simple ECC	Severe ECC	Maxillary ECC	p - value
Male	41 (50.6)	92 (50.0)	281 (50.1)	40 (51.3)*	
Female	40 (49.4)	92 (50.0)	280 (49.9)	38 (48.7)	p=0.997§

§ The value of p according to Hi square test.
* Absolute numbers and percentages in parentheses.

4.5.3. Association of the deft index with demographic characteristics

Table 4.5.3.1. presents the association of deft index with the demographic characteristics of the children involved in the study. It showed that there no significant statistical association with the gender of children and deft index was (p = 0.511), while the age of the children involved in the study proved to have a strong statistical link with deft index, where the older the children the higher was the deft index (p <0.001).

Table 4.5.3.1. Association of deft index with demographic characteristics, according to the General Linear Model.

Variable	Average value	95% CI	p - value
Gender:			
Male	6.5	6.2-6.9	p=0.511*
Female	6.4	6.0-6.8	
Age:			p<0.001 (2)‡
3 years	5.2	4.6-5.8	p<0.001
4 years	6.0	5.5-6.5	p<0.001
5 years	7.3	6.9-7.7	reference

* The value of p by general linear model.

‡ The total value of p and degrees of freedom are in parentheses.

4.5.4. Association of CI with demographic characteristics

Table 4.5.4.1. presents the Care Index connection with demographic characteristics of the children involved in the study. This connection based on the gender of the study subjects had no statistical significance (p = 0.200) with the CI. Also the age of the children involved in the study had no connection with CI index and it had no statistical significance (total value of p=0.301).

Table 4.5.4.1. Association of CI with demographic characteristics, according to the General Linear Model.

Variable	Average value	95% CI	p - value
Gender:			
Male	4.7	1.0-8.4	p=0.200*
Female	8.1	4.4-11.9	
Age:			p=0.301 (2)‡
3 years	52.0	1.8-102.2	p=0.887
4 years	17.2	6.5-40.9	p=0.467
5 years	35.2	21.8-48.6	reference

* The value of p by general linear model.

‡ The total value of p and degrees of freedom are in parentheses.

4.6. Socio-economic characteristics of the study subjects

4.6.1. Distribution of subjects according to socio-economic characteristics

Table 4.6.1.1. shows the distribution of study subjects according to their socio-economic characteristics. From the reported data it appears that most of the children had mothers with higher education (40.8%), followed by 33% of children whose mothers had a secondary education, compared with only 3% of children, whose mothers had elementary level education and about 14% of children had mothers with postgraduate education.

Regarding the income level, the respective families of children who were involved in the study, it was observed that most of them, that is, about 80% had an average income level, compared with 11% who reported low levels of income and 9.5% had higher income levels.

Table 4.6.1.1. Subject distribution based on SES.

Variable	Number	Percentage
Mother's education:		
Elementary	28	3.1
Middle school	85	9.4
High school	298	33.0
College	369	40.8
Postgraduate	124	13.7
Income level:		
Low	102	11.3
Average	716	79.2
High	86	9.5

4.6.2. Distribution of ECC by socio-economic characteristics

Table 4.6.2.1. presents the ECC distribution by education level of mothers of children involved in the study, which noted that the severity of early childhood caries is lower in children whose mothers have higher levels of education (p <0.001).

Table 4.6.2.1. Distribution of ECC by mother's education in the study subjects.

Variable	No ECC	Simple ECC	Severe ECC	Maxillary ECC	p - value
Elementary	0 (0.0)	1 (0.7)	4 (1.0)	1 (0.9)*	
Middle school	0 (0.0)	1 (0.7)	21 (5.1)	0 (0.0)	
High school	7 (11.9)	27 (18.4)	158 (38.1)	26 (46.6)	
College	40 (67.8)	90 (61.2)	171 (41.2)	26 (46.6)	p<0.001§
Postgraduate	12 (20.3)	28 (19.0)	61 (14.7)	3 (5.4)	

§ The value of p according to Hi square test.
* Absolute numbers and percentages in parentheses.

Table 4.6.2.2. reports that the higher the income level of the families of the children involved in the study, the lower the level of ECC and its severity (p <0.001).

Table 4.6.2.2. Distribution of ECC based on the income level of study subjects.

Variable	No ECC	Simple ECC	Severe ECC	Maxillary ECC	p – value
Elementary	3 (5.2)	8 (5.5)	73 (17.9)	3 (5.4)*	
High school	42 (72.4)	121 (82.9)	308 (75.7)	48 (85.7)	p<0.001§
College	13 (22.4)	17 (11.6)	26 (6.4)	5 (8.9)	

§ The value of p according to Hi square test.
* Absolute numbers and percentages in parentheses.

4.6.3. Association of deft index with socio-economic characteristics

Table 4.6.3.1. represents the association of deft index with socio-economic characteristics in the families of children involved in the study. It was noted that the educational level of the mother and family income level had a statistically significant correlation with deft index (p <0.001).

Table 4.6.3.1. Association of deft index with socio-economic characteristics, according to the General Linear Model.

Variable	Average value	95% CI	p – value
Mother's education:			p<0.001 (4) ‡
Elementary	6.3	3.0-9.7	p=0.742*
Middle school	9.6	7.9-11.3	p<0.001
High school	7.9	7.2-8.4	p<0.001
College	5.9	5.1-6.0	p=0.727
Postgraduate	5.8	4.9-6.6	reference
Income level:			p<0.001 (2)
Low	9.3	8.5-10.2	p<0.001
Medium	6.2	5.9-6.6	p<0.001
High	4.3	3.3-5.4	reference

* The value of p by general linear model.
‡ The total value of p and degrees of freedom are in parentheses.

4.6.4. Association of Care Index with the socio -economic characteristics

Table 4.6.4.1. presents the association of the CI with the socio-economic characteristics in the children participating in the study. Maternal education is shown to have a statistically significant association in the overall CI value, in the children involved in the study. Focusing on the income level of the families of children participating in the study and CI correlation, it proved to have statistical significance (p = 0.018).

Table 4.6.4.1. Association of CI with socio-economic characteristics, according to the General Linear Model.

Variable	Average value	95% CI	p – value
Mother's education:			p=0.011 (4)‡
Elementary	2.4	30.8-35.6	p=0.617*
Middle school	17.1	10.2-34.5	p=0.541
High school	6.7	1.1-12.2	p=0.385
College	4.5	1.3-9.4	p=0.188
Postgraduate	11.1	2.6-19.6	reference
Income level:			p=0.018 (2)
Low	1.0	8.1-9.9	p=0.076
Medium	6.9	3.2-10.7	p=0.242
High	14.4	2.4-26.6	reference

* The value of p by general linear model.
‡ The total value of p and degrees of freedom are in parentheses.

4.7. Health features of study subjects

4.7.1. Distribution of subjects by health features

Table 4.7.1.1. shows the distribution of study subjects according to the characteristics of the general health situation in the children involved in the study. As regards the distribution of subjects by chronic diseases, it was noted that only 3.4% were suffering from some form of chronic disease, compared with 97% who had no health problems associated with chronic diseases. About 2.5% of children participating in the study received continuous treatment and almost 53% of children receive vitamin and mineral supplements on a regular basis. Based on the birth weight of children participating in the study our research showed that only 6% of all children involved in this study were born weighing less than 2500 grams, compared to 97% of those who at birth had a weight greater or equal to 2,500 grams.

Table 4.7.1.1. Distribution of study subjects by health features.

Variable	Number	Percentage
Chronic disease:		
Yes	31	3.4
No	873	96.6
Regular treatment:		
Yes	22	2.4
No	882	97.6
Vitamin & mineral supplements:		
Yes	475	52.5
No	429	47.5
Child's birth weight:		
<2500 gr.	55	6.1
≥2500 gr.	849	93.9

4.7.2. ECC Distribution the according to health features

Table 4.7.2.1. presents ECC distribution based on the presence of chronic diseases in children participating in the study. Based on data analysis we were able to conclude that there is no significant statistical correlation between the chronic diseases (association) and early childhood caries.

Table 4.7.2.1. ECC distribution by chronic disease in the study subjects.

Variable	No ECC	With ECC	p - value
Chronic disease: Yes	0 (0)*	31 (5.0)	
Chronic disease: No	59(100.0)	585 (95.0)	p=0.078§

§ The value of p according to Hi square test.
* Absolute numbers and percentages in parentheses.

Regular treatment received by children, who participated in the study, did not show any statistically significant association with ECC.

Table 4.7.2.2. ECC distribution based on the regular treatment received by study subjects.

Variable	No ECC	With ECC	p - value
Regular treatment: Yes	0 (0)*	22 (3.6)	
Regular treatment: No	59(100.0)	593 (96.4)	p=0.140§

§ The value of p according to Hi square test.
* Absolute numbers and percentages in parentheses.

Table 4.7.2.3. reports that severe cases of ECC are more pronounced in children who did not take vitamin and mineral supplements. In this case there was a statistically significant association (p <0.001).

Table 4.7.2.3. ECC Distribution by the intake of supplements, vitamins and minerals among the study subjects.

Variable	No ECC	Simple ECC	Severe ECC	Maxillary ECC	p - value
Supplements: yes	36 (12.5)*	75 (26.1)	147 (51.2)	29 (10.1)*	
Supplements: no	20 (6.3)	58 (18.2)	216 (67.9)	24 (7.5)	p<0.001§

§ The value of p according to Hi square test.
* Absolute numbers and percentages in parentheses.

Table 4.7.2.4. presents the distribution of ECC according to the birth weight of the child, which as the results showed had no statistical significant correlation (p = 0.184).

Table 4.7.2.4. ECC Distribution by birth weight among the study subjects

Variable	No ECC	Simple ECC	Severe ECC	Maxillary ECC	p - value
<2500 gr	2 (3.4)	4 (2.7)	30 (7.2)	4 (7.1)*	
≥2500 gr	57 (96.6)	143 (97.3)	384 (92.8)	52 (92.9)	p=0.184§

§ The value of p according to Hi square test.
* Absolute numbers and percentages in parentheses.

4.7.3. Association of deft index with health features

According to data reported by the study it appeared that there was a statistically significant association between deft index and chronic diseases present in children participating in the study as well as with the regular treatment they received (Table 4.7.3.1).

Table 4.7.3.1. The association of deft index with chronic diseases and regular treatment, based on the General Linear Model.

Variable	Average value	95% CI	p - value
Chronic disease:			
Yes	7.6	6.2-9.1	p<0.001*
No	6.4	6.1-6.8	
Regular treatment:			
Yes	6.4	6.0-6.7	p<0.001
No	3.1	1.3-4.9	

* The value of p by general linear model.

In Table 4.7.3.2. we noted that the deft index has a positive and statistically significant association with the intake of additional supplements by children in the study, but this association was weakened considerably in the case of the administration of vitamins during a periodical time frame.

Table 4.7.3.2. The association of deft index with vitamin and supplement intake, based on the General Linear Model.

Variable	Average value	95% CI	p - value
Supplements:			
Yes	5.5	4.9-5.9	p<0.001*
No	7.2	6.7-7.6	
Vitamins:			
Yes	6.3	5.8-6.8	p=0.145
No	6.0	2.1-14.1	

* The value of p by general linear model.

Table 4.7.3.3. represents the association of deft index with the child's birth weight. No statistically significant correlation was reported between them (p = 0,555), although the average value deft index is higher in children with birth weight <2500 g.

Table 4.7.3.3. Association of deft index with child's birth weight.

Variable	Average value	95% CI	p - value
Child's birth weight:			
<2500 gr.	6.9	5.5-8.2	p=0.555*
≥2500 gr.	6.5	6.1-6.8	

* The value of p by general linear model.

4.7.4. Association of Care Index with health features

The survey data showed a statistically significant association in the presence of chronic diseases and their regular treatment with the Care Index (Table 4.7.4.1).

Table 4.7.4.1. The association of CI with chronic diseases and their regular treatment, based on the General Linear Model.

Variable	Average value	95% CI	p – value
Chronic disease:			
Yes	11.9	2.8-26.5	p<0.001*
No	6.3	2.9-9.7	
Regular treatment:			
Yes	5.1	12.3-22.4	
No	6.7	3.3-10.1	p<0.001

* The value of p by general linear model.

Table 4.7.4.2. presents the connection between Care Index with the birth weight and vitamin and mineral supplements intake in children participating in the study. In analyzing the association between CI and weight of the child at birth, we found a statistically significant association (p = 0.001), as was the case of vitamin and mineral supplement intake which also showed a statistically significant association (p = 0.056).

Table 4.7.4.2. The association of CI with child's birth weight and supplement intake, based on the General Linear Model.

Variable	Average value	95% CI	p – value
Child's birth weight:			p=0.001*
<2500 gr.	23.1	9.9-36.2	p=0.011
≥2500 gr.	5.6	2.2-8.9	reference
Vitamin & mineral supplements:			p=0.056
Yes	9.8	4.3-15.2	p=0.190
No	4.9	0.1-9.8	reference

* The value of p by general linear model.

4.8. Characteristics of nutritional habits and use of sugars by the study subjects

4.8.1. Distribution the ECC by nutrition habits and the use of sugar

Table 4.8.1.1 reports the distribution of ECC by feeding habits of the children participating in the study where we observed an increasing trend of ECC as the result of the increase in the consumption of artificial foods and of the combined ones (p <0.001).

Table 4.8.1.1. ECC distribution according to nutritional habits in the study subjects.

Variable	No ECC	Simple ECC	Severe ECC	Maxillary ECC	p - value
Breastfed only	39 (11.3)	93 (26.9)	187 (54.0)	27 (7.8)*	
Artificial	8 (6.6)	22 (18.0)	77 (63.1)	15 (12.3)	p<0.001§
Combination	11 (5.5)	33 (16.4)	143 (71.1)	14 (7.0)	

§ The value of p according to Hi square test.
* Absolute numbers and percentages in parentheses by columns.

Table 4.8.1.2. presents the distribution of ECC by the time children who participated in the study stopped breastfeeding, and results showed that early childhood caries and its severity was more pronounced in children who had stopped breastfeeding after one year (p = 0.006).

Table 4.8.1.2. ECC distribution in study subjects, who stopped breastfeeding after the one year mark.

Variable	Simple ECC	Severe ECC	Maxillary ECC	p - value
Stopped breastfeeding after 1 year: yes	103 (76.3)	237 (63.4)	42 (77.8)*	
Stopped breastfeeding after 1 year: no	32 (23.7)	137 (36.6)	12 (22.2)	p=0.006§

§ The value of p according to Hi square test.
* Absolute numbers and percentages in parentheses.

Table 4.8.1.3. presents ECC distribution in children participating in the study, who used a bottle at night, demonstrating a statistically significant correlation (p <0.001).

Table 4.8.1.3. ECC distribution in the study subjects based on the bottle use during the night.

Variable	No ECC	Simple ECC	Severe ECC	Maxillary ECC	p - value
Pacifier at night: yes	10 (4.5)	24 (10.7)	171 (76.3)	19 (8.5)*	
Pacifier at night: no	45 (11.3)	107 (26.9)	213 (53.5)	33 (8.3)	p<0.001§

§ The value of p according to Hi square test.
* Absolute numbers and percentages in parentheses.

Table 4.8.1.4. reports the distribution of ECC based on the content of fruit juice in the bottle, and after the data analysis using the Hi Square test showed a statistically significant connection (association) (p <0.001) with an increasing tendency of more severe ECC among children who consumed fruit juice, compared to children who did not.

Table 4.8.1.4. ECC distribution in the study subjects, based on the content of fruit juice in the bottle used during the night.

Variable	No ECC	Simple ECC	Severe ECC	Maxillary ECC	p - value
Fruit juice: yes	8 (3.3)	42 (17.1)	175 (71.4)	20 (8.2)*	
Fruit juice: no	73 (11.1)	142 (21.5)	386 (58.6)	58 (8.8)	p<0.001§

§ The value of p according to Hi square test.
* Absolute numbers and percentages in parentheses by rows.

Table 4.8.1.5. describes ECC distribution based on the content of sweet tea in the bottle and it shows that severe ECC has an increasing tendency among children who consumed sweetened tea, compared to children who did not.

Table 4.8.1.5. ECC distribution in study subjects, based on the content of sweetened tea in the bottle used during the night.

Variable	No ECC	Simple ECC	Severe ECC	Maxillary ECC	p - value
Tea: yes	5 (3.8)	24 (18.3)	92 (70.2)	10 (7.6)*	
Tea: no	76 (9.8)	160 (20.7)	469 (60.7)	68 (8.8)	p=0.084§

§ The value of p according to Hi square test.
* Absolute numbers and percentages in parentheses.

Table 4.8.1.6. describes ECC distribution in children who consume lollipops, and after data processing was concluded it showed a statistically significant association (p<0.001) with an increasing tendency of severe ECC cases among children who consumed lollipops, compared to the children who did not.

Table 4.8.1.6. ECC distribution in study subjects, based on lollipop consumption.

Variable	No ECC	Simple ECC	Severe ECC	Maxillary ECC	p - value
Lollipop: yes	7 (12.8) *	44 (17.4)	186 (73.5)	16 (6.3)*	
Lollipop: no	52 (12.6)	99 (23.9)	225 (54.3)	38 (9.2)	p<0.001§

§ The value of p according to Hi square test.
* Absolute numbers and percentages in parentheses.

Table 4.8.1.7. presents the average age when the children involved in the study began to drink from a cup, which turned out to be about 17 months or 1.5 years. Also the average age when children started consuming solid foods was reported to be about the same as the age of onset of drinking from a cup, about 17.1 months.

Table 4.8.1.7. Average age when the children began to drink from a cup and started consuming solid foods.

Variable	Drinking from a cup	Solid foods
Age (month): *Average SD*	16.9 ± 8.9	17.1 ± 7.8

Table 4.8.1.8. presents the association of ECC with the age when children started drinking from a cup and results of the study show a statistically significant correlation (p = 0.008), demonstrating that children with ECC have a higher average age.

Table 4.8.1.8. The association of ECC with the average age when children started drinking from a cup, based on the General Linear Model.

Variable	Average age	95% CI	p – value
ECC:			
no	13.9	11.7-16.3	p=0.008*
yes	17.3	16.5-17.9	

* The value of p by general linear model.

Based on the association of ECC with the average age when children started consuming solid foods (Table 4.8.1.9.), results showed that children with ECC and those who showed no sign of ECC had approximately the same age (17 and 16.5 months respectively) a correlation of no statistical significance (p = 0.580).

Table 4.8.1.9. The association of ECC with the average age when children started consuming solid foods, based on the General Linear Model.

Variable	Average age	95% CI	p - value
ECC:			
no	16.5	14.4-18.5	p=0.580*
yes	17.1	16.4-17.7	

* The value of p by general linear model.

4.8.2. Association of deft index with eating habits and the use of sugars

Table 4.8.2.1. presents the association between the deft index and the child's eating habits, where statistical significance was reported.

Table 4.8.2.1. The association of deft index with nutrition habits.

Variable	Average value	95% CI	p - value
Nutrition habits:			
Breastfed only	5.9	5.5-6.4	
Formula milk	6.9	6.1-7.7	p<0.001*
Combination	7.1	6.5-7.7	

* The value of p by general linear model.

Table 4.8.2.2. presents a statistically significant correlation between deft index and duration of breastfeeding after age 1 year (p <0.001).

Table 4.8.2.2. The association of deft index with duration of breastfeeding.

Variable	Average value	95% CI	p – value
Breastfeeding after age 1 year:			
yes	5.9	5.6-6.4	p<0.001*
no	7.3	6.7-7.9	

* The value of p by general linear model.

Table 4.8.2.3. presents the connection of deft index with the use of baby bottle at night and its content. The data showed that there was a statistically significant assotiation between deft index and overnight baby bottle use (p <0.001). By focusing on the content of baby bottle, results showed that the content of the baby bottle with milk formula was borderline of statistical significance with deft index (p = 0.083), while this connection resulted very significant with regard to the content of fruit juice in bottle feeding (p <0.001).

Table 4.8.2.3. The association of deft index with the bottle use by at night and its contents.

Variable	Average value	95% CI	p - value
Bottle at night:			
yes	7.9	7.3-8.4	p<0.001*
no	5.8	5.3-6.1	
Bottle contents (formula milk):			
yes	6.8	6.3-7.3	p=0.083
no	6.3	5.9-6.6	
Bottle contents (fruit juice):			
yes	7.5	6.9-8.0	p<0.001
no	6.1	5.7-6.3	

Table 4.8.2.4. presents the association of deft index with the use of added sugar, in baby bottle, consumption of sugary products and lollipops by children involved in the study. The data showed that the use of sugar in children's diet has a statistically significant association (p <0.001) with deft index, as it was reported for the consumption of sugary products and lollipops, noting that the use of all these food products was closely related with the emergence of early childhood caries in children ages 3, 4 and 5 years old.

Table 4.8.2.4. The association of deft index with the use of added sugar in bottle, consumption of sugary products and lollipops, based on the General Linear Model.

Variable	Average value	95% CI	p - value
Added sugar in bottle:			
yes	9.6	8.9-10.4	p<0.001*
no	5.8	5.4-6.1	
Sugary products:			
yes	8.1	7.6-8.7	p<0.001
no	5.5	5.1-5.9	
Lollipop:			
yes	7.9	7.3-8.4	p<0.001
no	5.6	5.2-6.0	

* The value of p by general linear model.

Table 4.8.2.5 presents the correlation of deft index with the use of soothing pacifier and honey coated pacifier. The data showed that there was a statistically significant association between the use of the soothing pacifier and deft index (p = 0.015). Also there was a statistically significant association (p <0.001) between the deft index and the use of sugar / honey coated pacifier, thus highlighting the negative effects of sugar on the emergence of dental problems in children of preschool age.

Table 4.8.2.5. The association of deft index with the use of soothing pacifier and the pacifier coated with sugar/honey, based on the General Linear Model.

Variable	Average value	95% CI	p – value
Soothing pacifier:			
yes	7.0	6.5-7.6	p=0.015
no	6.1	5.7-6.6	
Pacifier coated with sugar/honey:			
yes	9.7	8.8-10.5	p<0.001*
no	5.7	5.4-6.1	

* The value of p by general linear model.

Table 4.8.2.6. presents the association between deft index and the average age of onset of use of solid foods where statistical significance was reported. Also this statistical significance was observed regarding the age when the child first starts drinking from a cup.

Table 4.8.2.6. The association between deft indexes with the age child starts solid foods

and the age he starts drinking from a cup, based on the General Linear Model.

Variable	Average value	95% CI	p – value
Age child starts solid foods (months)	17.02±7.8	5.5-7.1	p<0.001*
Age child starts drinking from cup (months)	16.9 ± 8.9	4.2-5.61	p<0.001

* The value of p by general linear model.

4.9. Oral hygiene characteristics in study subjects

4.9.1. ECC distribution based on the characteristics of oral hygiene

Table 4.9.1.1. presents ECC distribution by daily brushing teeth routine, which shows a statistically significant association (p <0.001) with an increasing trend of severe ECC among children who do not brush their teeth daily.

Table 4.9.1.1. ECC distribution in study subjects based on their daily tooth brushing routine.

Variable	No ECC	Simple ECC	Severe ECC	Maxillary ECC	p – value
Brushes teeth everyday: yes	49 (10.7)	110 (24.0)	259 (56.4)	41 (8.9)*	
Brushes teeth everyday: no	9 (4.2)	35 (16.3)	156 (72.6)	15 (7.0)	p<0.001§

§ The value of p according to Hi square test.
* Absolute numbers and percentages in parentheses.

Table 4.9.1.2. reports distribution of ECC by the frequency of brushing teeth, and shows a statistically significant association (p = 0.005) with an increasing trend of severe ECC among children who brush their teeth only once a day, comparing these data with children who brush their teeth two times a day.

Table 4.9.1.2. ECC distribution in the study subjects based on the frequency of their brushing.

Variable	No ECC	Simple ECC	Severe ECC	Maxillary ECC	p - value
Once a day	27 (5.9)	104 (22.7)	291 (63.5)	36 (7.9)*	
Twice a day	30 (15.3)	42 (21.4)	107 (54.6)	17 (8.7)	p=0.005§

§ The value of p according to Hi square test.
* Absolute numbers and percentages in parentheses.

Table 4.9.1.3. shows the distribution of ECC based on tooth brushing routine before bedtime by children involved in the study and there seems to be a statistically significant association (p<0.001) with an increasing trend of severe ECC among children who do not brush their teeth before bedtime, compared to children who regularly brush their teeth before bedtime.

Table 4.9.1.3. ECC distribution in study subjects based on their brushing routine before bedtime.

Variable	No ECC	Simple ECC	Severe ECC	Maxillary ECC	p - value
Brushes teeth before sleep: yes	51 (11.5)	101 (22.8)	253 (57.1)	38 (8.6)*	
Brushes teeth before sleep: no	8 (3.5)	43 (19.0)	159 (70.4)	16 (7.1)	p<0.001§

§ The value of p according to Hi square test.
* Absolute numbers and percentages in parentheses.

4.9.2. Association of deft index with oral hygiene features

Table 4.9.2.1. presents the average age when the children involved in the study, started to brush their teeth for the first time which was about 29 months or 2.4 years. This table also shows the connection of the deft index with the age children started to brush their teeth, which as shown by data is statistically significant (p = 0.003), respectively, demonstrating clearly that the later the tooth brushing routine starts the more dental problems will be present in children. Also, the frequency of tooth brushing and their bedtime brushing routine have resulted in a statistically significant correlation with the deft index (p <0.001).

Table 4.9.2.1. The association between deft indexes and the age child starts brushing and the frequency of tooth brushing, based on the General Linear Model.

Variable	Average value	95% CI	p – value
Age child starts brushing teeth (months)	29.02±10.3	0.01-0.08	p=0.003*
Brushes teeth everyday:			
yes	5.9	5.5-6.3	p<0.001
no	7.7	7.1-8.2	
How many times brushes teeth:			
Once a day	6.7	6.3-7.1	p<0.001
Twice a day	5.8	5.2-6.4	
Brushes teeth before bed:			
yes	5.9	5.4-6.2	p<0.001
no	7.7	7.1-8.2	

* The value of p by general linear model.

Table 4.9.2.2. presents the association of deft index when brushing teeth deft assisted by a parent, which in total estimated value of the general linear model have resulted in statistically significant.

Table 4.9.2.2. The association of the deft index with the person who brushes child's teeth, based on the General Linear Model.

Variable	Average value	95% CI	p – value
Who brushes child's teeth:			
			p<0.001(2) ‡
Child himself	7.4	6.9-7.9	p=0.003*
Parent	5.3	4.6-5.9	p=0.036
Child and parent	6.2	5.6-6.8	reference

* The value of p by general linear model.
‡ The total value of p and degrees of freedom are in parentheses.

46

4.10. Oral care features in study subjects

4.10.1. ECC distribution based on oral care features

Table 4.10.1.1. presents the average age when children involved in the study have completed their first visit to the dentist, age which is reported to be relatively high at around 42 months or almost 3.5 years.

Table 4.10.1.1. Average age when children paid their first visit to dentist.

Variable	First visit to dentist
Age (months): *Average SD*	41.6 ± 13.2

Table 4.10.1.2. presents the correlation between the average age of the child's first visit to the dentist with early childhood caries. Results show that children with ECC cases had higher average age for their first dentist visit (42.2 months or 3.5 years) than children without any signs of ECC (36 months to 3 years), a correlation of statistical significance (p = 0.025).

Table 4.10.1.2. The association of ECC with the average age of child's first visit to the dentist, based on the General Linear Model.

Variable	Average age	95% CI	$p-value$
ECC:			
no	36.0	30.8-41.1	p=0.025*
yes	42.2	40.6-43.7	

*Value of p according to general linear model

Table 4.10.1.3. presents sealed teeth in children involved in the study, the absolute number, the average and standard deviation, and minimum and maximum value.

Table 4.10.1.3. Sealed teeth in the study subjects.

Number	904
Average	0.09
Standard Deviation	0.593
Minimum	0
Maximum	6

Table 4.10.1.4. presents in detail the distribution of children's sealed teeth in absolute numbers and their respective percentages.

Table 4.10.1.4. Distribution of sealed teeth in study subjects.

Variable	Number	Percentage
Sealed teeth:		
No sealed teeth	876	96.9
1 sealed teeth	6	0.7
2 sealed teeth	4	0.4
3 sealed teeth	9	1.0
4 sealed teeth	4	0.4
5 sealed teeth	2	0.2
6 sealed teeth	3	0.3

Table 4.10.1.5. reflects the distribution of ECC by placement of sealants by a dentist, in children participating in the study, which clearly shows that there is no statistically significant association (p = 0.115) between severe ECC and placement of sealants by the dentist, although the number of children with ECC (in absolute numbers and percentage), who did not have any sealants placed, is higher than the number of children with ECC who had their teeth coated with sealants.

Table 4.10.1.5. ECC distribution in study subjects based on the sealant placement.

Variable	No ECC	Simple ECC	Severe ECC	Maxillary ECC	p - value
Sealant: yes	4 (12.1)*	12 (36.4)	16 (48.5)	1 (3.0)	
Sealant: no	54 (8.7)	130 (20.9)	383 (61.7)	54 (8.7)	p=0.115§

§ The value of p according to Hi square test.
* Absolute numbers and percentages in parentheses.

Table 4.10.1.6. shows the distribution of ECC by fluoridation of the teeth of the children involved in the study and which has a statistically significant association (p = 0.010) with the trend of increased severe ECC among children who do not perform fluoridation of the teeth, compared with children who had their fluoridation done by a dentist dentist.

Table 4.10.1.6. ECC distribution in study subjects based on fluoridation process.

Variable	No ECC	Simple ECC	Severe ECC	Maxillary ECC	p - value
Fluoridation: yes	11 (15.9)	22 (31.9)	33 (47.8)	3 (4.3)*	
Fluoridation: no	46 (8.0)	121 (21.0)	357 (61.9)	53 (9.2)	p=0.010§

§ The value of p according to Hi square test.
* Absolute numbers and percentages in parentheses.

4.10.2. Association of deft index with oral care habits

Table 4.10.2.1. presents the association of deft index with the age when the child has completed his first visit to the dentist, which showed a statistically significant correlation ($p < 0.001$). While we observed no statistically significant correlation between the regular check-ups to the dentist and the deft index ($p = 0,747$), as was the case of fluoridation of the teeth of children by the dentist ($p = 0.320$), although the average value of deft index was higher among children who did not perform regular check-ups and dental fluorinations compared to other children, who had these procedures. While the placement of sealant by the dentist and deft index was reported to have a statistically significant association ($p = 0.045$)

Table 4.10.2.1. The association of deft index with regular check-ups, placement of sealants and fluoridation by dentists, based on the General Linear Model.

Variable	Average age	95% CI	p – value
Age of first visit to the dentist (months)	41.6 ± 13.2	4.01-7.3	p<0.001*
Regular check-ups to the dentist:			
yes	6.4	5.8-6.9	p=0.747
no	6.5	6.1-6.9	
Sealant placement:			
yes	4.9	3.5-6.5	p=0.045
no	6.5	6.2-6.9	
Fluoridation by dentist:			
yes	5.9	4.9-6.9	p=0.320
no	6.5	6.1-6.9	

*Value of p according to general linear model

Table 4.10.2.2. report the connection(association) of deft index with the use of fluoride supplements, which display a statistically significant association (p<0.001) between these factors.

Table 4.10.2.2. The association of deft index with fluoride supplement intake by children, based on the General Linear Model.

Variable	Average age	95% CI	$p - value$
Fluoride supplements :			
yes	4.5	3.8-5.2	p<0.001*
no	6.8	6.5-7.1	

*Value of p according to general linear model

5. DISCUSSION

5.1. The prevalence of Early Childhood Caries (ECC)

The results of our study reported that the prevalence of early childhood caries in children 3-5 years in public kindergartens in Tirana was 91%, a value that is very high considering that Tirana is the capital city of Albania.

Various authors report that the prevalence of caries in preschool has declined in most of the developed countries (24, 25), but in developing countries and even some developed countries there is a growing trend (26, 27). Conclusions based on the results from these studies show that early childhood caries is considered an epidemic in developing countries (48). Increasing urbanization and the rapid changes related to eating habits are probably the factors that contribute most to the deterioration of dental health in developing countries (22).

In a recent survey of the literature review conducted by the authors in 2013, important data was extracted, data obtained from various studies regarding the prevalence of early childhood caries and deft index (140). The maximum age of the children involved in these studies, selected for review is 5 years which coincides with the maximum age of children part of our study. A closer look at the literature review showed that the prevalence of ECC has a very big margin in various places ranging from 17 to 94%. (140).

Meanwhile, a study done in Kastriot municipality in Kosovo showed that the prevalence of ECC in children 3-5 years was 25% and the dmft index was 12.5 (141).

These comparative data, including the data from our study, are presented in detail in Table 5.2.1.1.

Table 5.2.1.1. Prevalence of e ECC and dmft/deft index in several studies.

Study (authors, year)	Place (city, country)	No. of children	Age (years)	% (deft>0)	dmft/deft (avg. value)
Mantonanaki et al. (2013)	Attica (Greece)	605	5	17	3.23
Ferro et al. (2006)	Veneto (Italy)	290	5	27	1.34
Mora et al. (2000)	Granada (Spain)	173	2 – 3	37	3.52
Pitts et al. (2007)	Scotland (UK)	11161	5	46	2.16
Wigen et al. (2011)	Oslo (Norwegian)	1348	5	11	1.4
Ferreira et al. (2007)	Canoas (Brazil)	1487	0 – 5	40	1.53
Simratvir et al. (2009)	Ludhiana (India)	609	3 – 5	59	4.76
Sufia et al. (1974)	Lahore (Pakistan)	700	3 – 5	75	1.85
Autio-Gold et al. (2005)	Florida (USA)	221	5	48	2.5
Wanjau et al. (2006)	Philadelphia (USA)	269	5	53	2.18
Li et al. (2012)	Shanghai (China)	1850	5	64	2.96
Cleaton-Jones et al. (2008)	Johannesburg (South Africa)	7185	2 – 5	59	3.4
Cariño et al. (2003)	Northern Philippines (Philippines)	448	5	**94**	**9.8**
Begzati-Rexhepi et al. (2012)	Kastriot (Kosovo)	108	3 – 5	25	**12.5**
Petro. E. (2015)	Tirana (Albania)	904	3-5	**91**	**6.45**

As observed by the comparative data offered by the literature, the prevalence of ECC in our study (91%) is slightly lower than the prevalence of ECC in the Philippines (94%), but this is a much higher figure than most authors present in their studies, including neighboring countries like Kosovo, Italy and Greece. In Kastriot, Kosovo the study was conducted in one of the municipalities with the lowest income level and the 25% figure of the prevalence of ECC in this municipality is much smaller than that reported in our study.

In addition to the alarming prevalence figure, most of the children involved our study (62.1%) suffer severe form of the ECC indicating greater severity of early childhood caries.

5.2. deft index

The results of our study show that the average value of the deft index is 6.45, while average values for individual dt, et and ft indexes are respectively 6.2, 0.07 and 0.2. Comparative data from the literature, presented in the above table 5.2.1.1, show that the deft index in our study is a much higher figure than in the majority of studies carried out by various authors, with the exception of Philippines which has a higher deft index i value (9.8) and Kosovo which has a dmft index much higher (12.5) nearly double the value of our index.

5.3. Care Index (CI)

The results of our study show that the average value of CI is 3.1%. This index provides data indicating that only 3.1% of the decayed deciduous teeth were treated by a dentist and the majority is untreated. This shows a very low level of dental care for children involved in the study. This figure is lower than the results of a study conducted in South Africa where the level of care was only 20% and the majority of children 4-5 years old had ECC untreated by the public service or the private one (101).

5.4. Demographic factors

Results of this study showed that about 20% of the children were age 3 years, 34% were 4 years old and 46% were of age 5 years. The highest percentage of children was of age 5 as a result of higher enrollment of these children in kindergartens and their lower rejection rates during the examination process. Regarding gender distribution can say that the representation of male / female population balance was almost complete.

Results of our study showed that age is a significant factor because as the child grows ECC becomes more pronounced in all forms of its occurrence as reported in similar studies where the prevalence of ECC grows so significantly with the increasing age (42, 142, 143). According to different authors this can be explained as increased exposure to cariogenic factors over time, the lack of a timely first visit and preventive measures which should be carried out immediately after the teeth have erupted (12, 13, 32, 118, 123, 144). Compared with the results of a study conducted in nurseries in Tirana in 2010, the prevalence of ECC was in lower numbers (47%) of children at a younger age, 1-3 years old (49).

With regard to the gender of the children participating in our study no statistical association was reported, both males and females are affected to the same extent from early childhood caries. Also, no statistically significant association was reported between the gender of the child and the deft index, while the age of the children involved in the study proved have a strong statistical correlation with deft index, where the older the children were, the higher was the deft index as reported in the literature studies (25).

5.5. Social - economic factors

Most of the children involved in this study had mothers with higher education (40.8%), followed by 33% of children whose mothers had a high school education, compared with only 3% of children, whose mothers had elementary level education and about 14% of children had mothers with postgraduate education. Regarding the income level in the families of children who were included in the study, we noted that most of them, that is, about 80% had an average income level, compared to 11% who reported low levels of income and 9.5% who had higher income level.

Educational level and economic factors are significant factors, as the results of our study reported the prevalence and severity of dental early childhood caries is lower in children whose mothers have a higher educational level and whose families have higher income. It was also noted that the mother's education level and family's economic status have demonstrated a statistically significant correlation with the deft index which was lower in children with higher socio-economic status. These data match the literature studies that show a close association between socio-economic status and early childhood caries (43, 47, 54, 68, 71, and 74). The high level of education is closely related to the low prevalence of ECC (144).

Also this study reported a statistical significance between the family socio-economic status and Care Index which means that the level of care is lower in children living in households with lower education and lower income. The low educational level of the mother affects the lack of information and oral health care for children (43, 71, 73). Also, mothers with lower educational level are unmotivated to participate in prevention programs and receive information about oral health (144). Also parents with low income level have social and financial disadvantages that reduce their ability to live in a healthy environment and get professional quality service. These individuals are likely to neglect oral health problems, the need for care and prevention for themselves and their children (68, 73, 74, 75, and 144). This should motivate us to think of better opportunities that should be offered to children of preschool age, who live in households with lower income level, to secure them better access to public dental service.

5.6. Health factors

Results of this study showed that only 3.4% of children suffered any chronic diseases, compared to the majority, about 97% who had no health problems. About 2.5% of children participating in the study received regular medication and almost 53% of children receive vitamin and mineral supplements on a regular basis with. The birth weight of children participating in the study showed that only 6% of all children included in this study were born weighing less than 2500 grams, and in the majority of children (97%) the birth weight was greater or equal to 2,500 grams, a weight that is considered normal according to WHO criteria (145).

The results of our study showed that the presence of chronic diseases and their regular treatment had a statistically significant association with early childhood caries and deft index as reported in the literature (146). Also the same connection was observed with Care Index, which means that these children are at greater risk from the ECC, but they take better care for the treatment of early childhood caries.

Our results indicate that severe ECC is more pronounced in children who did not take additional supplements and this represents a statistically significant association not only with the spread of the ECC but also with deft index or Care Index. These results are similar to the literature data, confirming that taking additional supplements affect the prevention and control of early childhood caries (147, 148).

The results of this study did not observe a carrelation between the ECC and birth weight, as reported in a study by author Shulman in 2005 (149). Also no statistically significant correlation was reported between the deft index and weight of the child at birth, although the average deft index value is higher in children with birth weight <2500 g. Similar data have been reported in some of the literature, but the correlation observed was statistically significant only due to the presence of mineralization of enamel defects and the role of birth complications in the subsequent development of enamel (150, 151). This discrepancy with the data presented by our study is believed to be the result of the uneven distribution of the sample subjects in our study in association with birth weight, as only a very small number of children (6%) had a birth weight <2500 g . While a statistically significant association was observed between the Care Index and the child's birth weight, which means that parents care more for these children as a result of greater fear for their health from birth.

5.7. Nutritional habits

The results of our study refer to a strong statistical association between the feeding habits of the children participating in the study and early childhood caries, where we observed an increasing trend of ECC due to consumption of artificial food or the combined ones. Also, a strong statistical correlation was found between the deft index and feeding habits, where the deft index is lower in breastfed children. According to WHO recommendations, in addition to other positive effects on child's health, breast milk influences and prevents ECC (152).

Also, it results that early childhood caries and its severity is more pronounced in children who had stopped breastfeeding after a year. As several other authors conclude breastfeeding or prolonged breastfeeding is not the cause of ECC (77, 147). These results comply with the recommendations of WHO to promote breastfeeding for infants up to 24 months (152). Meanwhile, in our study there was a significant association between the deft index and prolonged breastfeeding, where the deft index was higher in children who did not stop breastfeeding after the first year. This contradiction present also in our study is one of the most controversial issues today, and many opinions exist on the subject, opinions that contradict each other, based on opposite results received by various studies of the literature relating to this topic (22, 153). The bad habits of feeding are thought to be the cause, and although breast milk is very important for ensuring best nutrition babies, frequent feedings, especially at night when the child's teeth have already erupted, can affect presence of ECC (56). Breast milk is not cariogenic food, but it contains lactose which increases the affinity of the cariogenic bacteria in the oral cavity and allows them to settle on the surface of the tooth. As the result of the effect of these bacteria the lactose ferments and causes the demineralization of enamel. After frequent use of lactose or breast milk, the production of acid in the dental plaque increases (21).Higher caries experienced among children who were breastfed over one year old, is the result of mother's availability, she is present whenever the child wants to feed, throughout the day, but also because mothers use breastfeeding throughout the night to put the child to sleep or to calm a crying child (61).

Also, another aspect that reflects the wrong methods applied during breastfeeding is the constant contact for a prolonged, especially during sleep. Constant sucking of the bottle content through the night directly affects the emergence of ECC due to the decrease of salivary flux and deposit of carbohydrates in the oral cavity (7). Results of our study observed statistically significant association between the distribution of ECC and the use of a night bottle by children participating in the study, also we observed a statistically significant association between the deft index and bottle use at night. These results reinforce the opinion expressed by many authors that the use of the bottle at night increases the risk for ECC much more than bottlefeeding itself if this would be appropriately done (21, 90, 118, 137, 154).

The use of "calming" bottle, coated with sugar or honey is absorbed by young children to calm their crying or before sleep is a risk factor for the emergence of ECC (53). Our study results showed a statistically significant association between the use of "soothing" bottle, coated with sugar / honey and the deft index, noting that the use of sugar additives is closely related to cavities early childhood confirming again the wrong methods for the use of "soothing" bottle.

Fruit juices and sugary drinks aid in the emergence of early childhood caries because they have an added sweetening agent, usually fructose that increases their acid reaction. Fruit juices and sugary drinks cause a significant decrease in pH of the plate (21). When these are used by the children who display signs of ECC, the enamel erosion ECC progresses rapidly and spreads in a more aggressive form considered "rampant caries" (9).Our study reported a statistically significant association between the content of fruit juice or tea in the bottle and ECC, results show an increasing trend of severe ECC among children who consume fruit juice or tea, compared with children who did not consume them. Also, the results showed that the content of the baby bottle with milk formula was at the border of statistical significance with the deft index, while this connection was very significant when considering the content of fruit juice and tea, which means that in compared to milk formula, with no sugary additions, sugary drinks are one of the most dangerous factors that contribute to the emergence of ECC.

Sucrose is the carbohydrate with the highest cariogenic effect and consumption of carbohydrates in liquid form is a risk factor that affects the emergence of the ECC due to prolonged contact with the surface of the tooth (8, 53, 55). Maxillary anterior caries prevalence is higher in children who use the bottle with sweetened milk or other sugary drinks, than in children who use a bottle of milk without added sugar or water (7). Results of this study showed that the use of added sugar in the milk bottle has a significant statistical link with deft index, as it was also reported for the consumption of sugary products and lollipops. In terms of lollipop consumption, children in this study showed a statistically significant association with the growing trend of severe ECC among children who consume them, compared with children who don't. These results highlighted the negative effects of sugary products in the emergence of dental problems in children of preschool age.

The average age when children in the study started to drink from a cup, was about 17 months or 1.5 years. Also the average age when children started consuming solid foods was reported to be about the same as the age of onset of use of glass, about 17.1 months, while the literature recommends the use of the cup after the age of 6 months and the use of solid food after 12 months (21, 154). In our study the connection of ECC with the age when children began drinking from a cup was statistically significant, demonstrating that children with ECC started to drink from a cup later than children who had no signs of ECC. Also this statistical significance was observed in association with deft index. While children with ECC as well as children without ECC had an approximately similar age for the consumption of solid foods and there was no statistically significant link between the average age of the onset of feeding solids and ECC or deft, which can be explained by the impact of other major factors.

5.8. Oral hygiene

The literature suggests that the application of methods of oral hygiene for children should start to as soon as the first tooth erupts, brushing teeth with a tooth brush should begin at age 2 and at 3 years old the child should start using fluorinated toothpaste which is the local method with lower cost and higher efficiency in the prevention of ECC and the most widespread method that can be widely used by all children (89, 120, 122, 123). But in this age child cannot carry out an efficient cleaning himself and so the brushing of teeth should be assisted by a parent (81, 155).

The results showed that the average age when the children i in this study begun brushing their teeth for the first time is at about 29 months, or 2.4 years, not far from the suggested age and in literature (143). The results also showed that there is a link between the deft index and the age when children are started to brush their teeth for the first time, which statistically significant, namely reporting that the latter the child starts brushing the teeth, the higher was the caries experience of the children in this study. In accordance with the results of various authors, our study showed that association deft index, when brushing was assisted by parent, is statistically significant with a lower index in this case. Parents, especially mothers play an important role not only in facilitating the procedure of brushing, but also in teaching the fundamentals of oral hygiene care (79, 83, 84).

Deciduous tooth surfaces must be carefully cleaned after each meal (10). An important factor affecting milk protect teeth from caries early childhood is regular brushing teeth daily with fluorinated toothpaste, especially in the evening before bedtime (54, 113). According to the AAPD frequency of brushing teeth, to reduce the risk of ECC in children, it is recommended 2 times a day (97).

Results of our study showed that there is a statistically significant association with the growing trend of severe ECC among children who do not brush their teeth every day. The same results were reported for children who brush their teeth only once a day, compared to children who brush their teeth two times a day; as well as for children who do not brush their teeth before bedtime, compared with children who perform dental brushing before bedtime. Also daily tooth brushing, frequency of brushing before bedtime have resulted in statistically significant association with deft index which means that children who properly implement the rules of oral hygiene have a lower caries experience.

5.9. Oral Health Care

According to the recommendations of AAPD and ADA, which are also supported by different authors, the first visit to the dentist should be as soon as the child's first tooth grows and no later than age 1 year (96, 97, 98, 156, 157, 158, 159).This way, the parent has the opportunity to be informed of the proper way of breastfeeding and bottle feeding, the role of carbohydrates, oral hygiene care, methods of fluoridation and sealant placement. The results showed that the average age when children in our study paid their first visit to the dentist is relatively high, about 42 months or almost 3.5 years, but is lower compared to the data obtained from a study conducted in our country in 2009 which showed that the average age of the first visit to the dentist for children was 7 years and the main reason for this delay, in 98% of cases, was the fear that the parents themselves had experienced from their first meeting with the dentist. Also the 2009 study showed that out of the 301 parents interviewed, only 12% of them had taken the child for the first visit to the dental cabinet no later than age 1 year (88). In our study the association between ECC and the average age when the children went to the dentist for their first check had a statistical significance, which means that children with ECC had higher average age than children without ECC. The results also showed a statistically significant association between deft index and age when the child had completed his first visit to the dentist, the later the first visit, the higher the number of early childhood caries.

All children must undergo periodic and continuous check-ups, every 6 months, while children with a high-risk for ECC should undergo periodic inspections 3-4 times a year (95, 96, 97, and 113). While our study did not observe any statistically significant association between periodic check-ups to the dentist and the deft index, the deft index average value was higher in children who did not have regular check-ups compared to other children who had their teeth regularly checked.

After eruption of the teeth in children prevention methods such as fluoridation of drinking water or fluoride supplements need to be applied (69, 122). Fluoridation of drinking water is a preventive systemic method that involves the whole community, but in recent decades this method has been less efficient in reducing the ECC due to the scarcity of fluorinated natural water resources which have become increasingly scarce and as a replacement they have been taking fluoride through other means such as those with local impact, through treatment in dental clinics (98, 109, 111, 120, 121, 160, 161).

Local prevention methods include fluoride mouth rinse aids, fluoride jellies and lacquers which are applied especially in children at high risk for early childhood caries. In developed countries these preventive measures are applied free by dental hygienists who perform periodic check-ups in preschool children (69, 115, 125, 160, 161). According to data obtained from the RHA (Regional Health Authority), there are no dentists / dental hygienist in kindergartens of Tirana, who could perform preventive procedures such as fluoridation. School doctors are available to perform occasional check-ups during the summer, at which time schools are closed. While the information we obtained in the kindergartens, part of our study, showed that no dentist from RHA had visited these kindergartens for a very long period of time.

Results of our study indicated a statistically significant association between ECC and fluoridation of children's teeth of children, and a growing trend of severe ECC among children who did not apply any fluoride treatment compared with children who had fluorinated teeth done by a dentist as recommended by literature data (115, 121, and 160). While we did not observe a statistically significant link between the fluoridation of teeth by a dentist and the deft index, although the average value of the deft index was higher among children who did not have fluorinations done by a dentist compared with other children, who had done it. Similar results are explained in the literature as a result of using combined methods fluoridation (toothpaste, solution, gel, spray) differing from the use of a single method (162).

This study reported the deft index association with the use of fluoride supplements, where a statistically significant association was observed between them, meaning that children who have taken fluoride supplements have less caries experiences. This coincides with data obtained from literature which recommend giving supplements of fluoride to children at high risk for ECC in doses carefully monitored by the dentist (26, 147, 148, 163, 164).

The application of sealants in the primary dental system is also another very important method of professional dental care. Until recently it was thought that sealants should be used only in permanent teeth, but today this procedure is recommended as a prophylactic measure effective in preventing caries spots and fissures in primary dentition especially in children at high risk of ECC (96, 97). According to the AAPD and ADA, retention of sealants in deciduous teeth is higher than in permanent teeth because at the time of sealant application temporary teeth have fully erupted and their crown is fully formed (96, 97, 130). Our results also indicated that the majority of children, 96.9% had no sealed tooth which means that most parents have not applied sealing of fissures in temporary teeth due to misinformation or lack of financial resources. While the association between ECC and placement of sealants by a dentist in children participating in this study, did not result in any statistically significant correlation, the number of children with severe ECC (in absolute and percentage), who had not any sealants placed was bigger than the number of those who had sealants placed. While the link between placement of sealants by a dentist and deft index had a statistically significant association. These results match with the data in the literature reporting that the sealed primary teeth are less affected by early childhood caries, but the application of sealants should be combined with other methods of prevention and control ECC (131).

6. CONCLUSIONS

In conclusion of this study, based on data obtained from the results and cross- checking them with data from the literature on similar studies by various authors, we can draw the following conclusions:

1. This is the first study in our literature in the field of Pediatric Dentistry, which provides data on the prevalence of ECC and caries experience in primary teeth in children of preschool age (3-5 years) in the public kindergartens of the city of Tirana and which identifies factors associated with early childhood caries.

2. The prevalence of early childhood caries in children 3-5 years old in the public kindergartens of Tirana is very high (91%) and the majority of children (62.1%) suffer Severe ECC that indicates the gravity of this condition.

3. The average value of the deft index of 6.45 (SD ± 25.4) shows a high level of caries experience and the lower average value of the Care Index 3.1%, indicates a very low level of dental care in children with ECC.

4. Results of this study confirmed the association between the main risk factors and early childhood caries.

5. Parents lack the necessary information on proper nutrition, oral hygiene and oral health care for children in early childhood and thereafter.

6. In kindergartens of the city of Tirana no dentist from the Regional Health Authority has performed any check-ups in a very long period of time.

7. Preschool children, who live in households with low income levels, are not offered an opportunity to receiving better access to public dental service.

8. Designing ECC prevention strategies to address the community's needs is an urgent task for improving the oral health of preschool children in our country.

7. RECOMMENDATIONS

Recognizing the difficulties encountered in the treatment of children of preschool age, low access and the high cost of service, prevention of early childhood caries would be a more effective course of action than treatment. Based on the findings of this study we are able to suggest some recommendations for the prevention of ECC reducing the overall level of risk factors.

1. Strategies addressing the oral health of the community should be the responsibility of public health authorities and other government or non-governmental national organizations which should draft educational and informational programs to improve the oral health of preschool children in our country.

2. These programs should include parents, kindergarten and pre-school teachers, advisory personnel and pediatricians because all these groups are in frequent and continuous contact with the child.

3. Breastfeeding provides the best nutrition for infants, but if it continues after the age of 1 it should be limited, especially at night.

4. Contents of baby bottle should not have added sugar, honey or sugary juices and soothing bottle should not be coated with sugar / honey. Use of a bottle at night should be discontinued as soon as the first deciduous tooth erupts.

5. After the age of 6 months the child should start using a cup and after 1 year of age children should start consuming solid food.

6. Brushing teeth should begin at age 2 and it should be done by the parent / guardian. Brushing teeth should be done every day in the morning and evening with fluorinated toothpaste. In ECC high-risk cases fluoride solutions should be used daily or weekly.

7. Child's first visit to the dentist should be performed as soon as the first tooth erupts, no later than age 1 year and must be accompanied with continuous and periodic check-ups, depending on ECC risk, every 4 or 6 months.

8. Topical fluoride and fluoride supplements should be applied in children of preschool age in dosage and frequency prescribed and monitored very carefully by the dentist depending on the level of risk for ECC.

9. The application of sealants is also recommended as an effective prophylactic measure in preventing caries spots and fissures in primary dentition especially in children with high risk for early childhood caries.

10. For preschool children who live in households with low income level, they should be offered better opportunities for access to public dental service.

8. BIBLIOGRAPHY

1. Huntington NL, Kim J, Hughes ChV. Caries risk factors for Hispanic children affected by early childhood caries. Pediatric Dent 2002;24:536-542.
2. Ramos-Gomes FJ, Tomar SL, Ellison J, Artiga N, Sintes J, Vicuna G. Assessment of early childhood caries and dietary habits in a population of migrant Hispanic children in Stocken, California. ASDC J Dent Child 1999;66:395-403.
3. Schroth RJ, Moffatt ME. Determinants of early childhood caries in rural Mantoba community: a pilot study. Pediatr Dent 2005; 27(2): 114-20.
4. Belterami G. Les dents noires de tout-petits. Siècle Médical. In Belterami G (ed). La mélandontie infantile. Marseille: Leconte 1952.
5. Fass, Enl is bottle feeding of milk a factor in dental caries? J Dent Child 1962; 24: 245-51.
6. Tinanoff N. Introduction to early childhood caries conference: initial description and current understanding. Comm Dent Oral Epidemiol 1998; 26(Supplement 1): 5-7.
7. Reisine S, Douglass JM. Psychosocial and behavioural issues in early childhood caries. Comm Dent Oral Epidemiol 1998; 26(Supplement 1): 32-44.
8. Ripa LW. Nursing caries: A comprehensive review. Pediatr Dent 1988; 10: 268-282.
9. Seow WK. Biological mechanisms of early childhood caries. Comm Dent Oral Epidemiol 1998; 26(Supplement 1): 8-27.
10. TF, Horowity AM, Ismail AI, Maertens MP, Rozier RG, Selwity RH. Diagnosing and reporting early childhood caries for research purposes. J Public Health Dent 1999; 59: 129-7.
11. Gussy MG, Waters EG, Walsh O, Kilpatrick N. Early childhood caries: Current evidence for aetiology and prevention. Journal of Paediatrics and Child Health 2006; 42: 37-73.
12. American Academy of Pediatric Dentistry. Oral Health Policies. Pediatr. Dent. 2004; 26(7): 16-61.
13. Psoter WJ, Zhang H, Pendrys DG, Morse DE, Mayne ST. Classification of dental caries patterns in theprimary dentition: a multidimensional scaling analysis. Community Dent Oral Epidemiol 2003;31:231–238.
14. AAPD (American Academy of Pediatric Dentistry). Policy on Early Childhood Caries :classifications, consequences, and preventive strategies. 2008.
15. Kingman A, Selwitz RH. Proposed methods for improving the efficiency of the DMFS index in assessing initiation and progression of dental caries. Community Dent Oral Epidemiol 1997;25:60-68.
16. World Health Organization (WHO). A guide to oral health epidemiological investigations. Geneva: WHO 1979.
17. World Health Organization (WHO). Oral health surveys: Basic methods. 4th ed. Geneva: WHO 1997.
18. Ismail AI. Clinical diagnosis of precavitated carious lesions. Community Dent Oral Epidemiol 1997;25:13-23.
19. Pitts NB. Diagnostic tools and measurements, impact on appropriate care. Community Dent Oral Epidemiol 1997;25:24-35.

20. Roshi E, Burazeri G. Epidemiologjia. 2008;4: 78-81.
21. Du M, Bian Z, Guo L. Caries patterns and their relationship to infant feeding and socio-economic status in 2-4 year old Chinese children. International Dental Journal 2000; 50: 385-389.
22. Maupomé G. An introspective qualitative report on dietary patterns and elevated levels of dental decay in a deprived urban population in Northern Mexico. J Dent Childr 1998; 276-285.
23. World Health Organization (WHO, 2007a).
24. Nordblad A, Souminen-Taipale L, Rasilainen J, Karhunen T. Suun (Oral Health Care at Health Centers from the 1970s to the year 2000). Helsinki: National Research and Development Center for Welfare and Health (STAKES), Report 278, 2004.
25. Holm AK. Caries in the preschool child: international trends. J Dent 1990;18:291-295.
26. Center for Disease Control (CDC). Oral health improving for most Americans, but tooth decay among preschool children on the rise. Centers for Disease Control and Prevention. (2007).
27. Pitts NB, Palmer JD. The dental caries experience of 5-year-old children in Great Britain. Surveys coordinated by the British Association for the Study of Community Dentistry in 1993/94. Community Dent Health 1995;12:52-58.
28. Milnes AR. Description and epidemiology of nursing caries. J Public Health Dent 1996;56:38-50.
29. Douglass JM, Tinanoff N, Tang JM, Altman DS. Dental caries patterns and oral health behaviors in Arizona infants and toddlers. Community Dent Oral Epidemiol 2001;29:14-22.
30. Douglass JM, Wei Y, Zhang BX, Tinanoff N. Caries prevalence and patterns in 3-6-year-old Beijing children. Community Dent Oral Epidemiol 1995;23:340-343.
31. Szatko F, Wierzbicka M, Dybizbanska E, Struzycka I, Iwanicka-Frankowska E. Oral health of Polish three-year-olds and mothers' oral health-related knowledge. Community Dent Health 2004;21:175-180.
32. Berkowitz RJ. Causes, treatment and prevention of early childhood caries; A microbiologic perspective. J Can Dent Assoc 2003;69:304-307.
33. Tang JM, Altamn DS, Robertson DC, O'Sullivan DM, Douglas JM, Tinanoff N. Dental caries prevalence and treatment levels in Arizona preschool children. Public Health Rep 1997;112:319-329.
34. O'Sullivan DM, Douglass JM, Champany R, Eberling S, Tetrev S, Tinanoff N. Dental caries prevalence and treatment among Navajo preschool children. J Public Health Dent 1994 ;54:139-144.
35. Rosenblatt A, Zarzar P. The prevalence of early childhood caries in 12- to 36-month-old children in Recife, Brazil. ASDC J Dent Child 2002;69:319-324.
36. Peressini S, Leake JL, Mayhall JT, Maar M, Trudeau R. Prevalence of early childhood caries among First Nations children, District of Manitoulin, Ontario. Int J Paediatr Dent 2004;14:101-110.
37. Jin BH, Ma DS, Moon HS, Paik DI, Hahn SH, Horowitz AM. Early childhood caries: prevalence and risk factors in Seoul, Korea. J Public Health Dent 2003;63:183-188.
38. Fujiwara T, Sasada E, Mima N, Ooshima T. Caries prevalence and salivary mutans streptococci in 0-2-year-old children of Japan. Community Dent Oral Epidemiol 1991;19:151-154.

39. Carino KMG, Shinida K, Kawaguchi Y. Early childhood caries in northern Philippines. Community Dent Oral Epidemiol 2003;31:81-89.
40. Mayanagi H, Saito T, Kamiyama K. Cross-sectional comparisons of caries time trends in nursery school children in Sendai, Japan. Community Dent Oral Epidemiol 1995;23:344-349.
41. Tsai AI, Chen CY, Li LA, Hsiang CL, Hsu KH. Risk indicators for early childhood caries in Taiwan. Community Dent Oral Epidemiol 2006;34:437-445.
42. Jose B, King NM. Early childhood caries lesions in preschool children in Kerala, India. Pediatr Dent 2003;25:594-600.
43. Al-Hosani E, Rugg-Gunn A. Combination of low parental educational attainment and high parental income related to high caries experience in pre-school children in Abu Dhabi. Community Dent Oral Epidemiol 1998;26:31-36.
44. Al-Malik MI, Holt RD, Bedi R. The relationship between erosion, caries and rampant caries and dietary habits in preschool children in Saudi Arabia. Int J Paediatr Dent 2001;11:430-439.
45. Rajab LD, Hamdan MA. Early childhood caries and risk factors in Jordan. Community Dent Health 2002;19:224-229.
46. Kiwanuka SN, Astrom AN, Trovik TA. Dental caries experience and its relationship to social and behavioural factors among 3-5-year-old children in Uganda. Int J Paediatr Dent 2004;14:336-346.
47. Masiga MA, Holt RD. The prevalence of dental caries and gingivitis and their relationship to social class amongst nursery-school children in Nairobi, Kenya. Int J Paediatr Dent 1993;3:135-140.
48. Weinstein P, Domoto P, Koday M, Leroux B. Results of a promising open trial to prevent baby bottle tooth decay: a fluoride varnish study. ASDC J Dent Child 1994;61:338-341.
49. Kelmendi M, Gace E. Kariesi i femijerise se hershme, studim epidemiologjik. 2010; referim ne Konferencen XVI Kombetare Dentare Shqiptare.
50. Nunn JH, Welbury RR, Gordon PH, Stretton-Downes S, Green-Abate C. Dental health of children in an integrated urban development programme for destitute mothers with twins in Addis Ababa. Int Dent Journal 1992; 42(6): 445-450.
51. Tinanoff N, O'Sullivan DM. Early childhood caries: overview and recent findings. Pediatr Dent 1997; 19: 12-16.
52. Lamis D, Hamdan MAM. Early childhood caries and risk factors in Jordan. Community Dental Health 2002; 19: 224-229.
53. Dimitrova MM, Kukleva MP, Kordeva VK. Prevalence of early childhood caries and risk factors in children from 1 to 3 years of age in Plovdiv, Bulgaria. Folia Med (Plovdiv) 2002; 44(1): 60-3.
54. Savegh A, Dini EL, Holt RD, Bedi R. Oral health, sociodemographic factors, dietary and oral hygiene practices in Jordanian children. J Dent 2005; (3395): 379-88.
55. Jamel H, Plaschaert A, Sheiham A. Dental caries experience and availability of sugars in Iraqi children before and after the United Nations Sanctions. Int Dent J 2004; 54(1): 21-5.
56. Erickson PR, Mazhari E. Investigation of the role of human breast milk in caries development. Am Acad Ped Dent 1999; 21(2): 86-90.
57. Goepferd SJ. Infant oral health: a rationale. J Dent Childr 1986; July/Aug: 257-260.
58. Ayhan H. Influencing factors of nursing caries. J Clin Pediatr Dent 1996; 20(4): 313-315.

59. Newburn, E. Dental caries in the future: a global view. Proc Finn Dent So 1992; 88(3-4): 155-61.
60. Petro E, Brovina D. Transmetimi vertikal i Streptokokut Mutans ne Kariesin e Femijerise se Hershme. Revista Shkencore Stomatologjike APOLONIA 2014; 31:21-28.
61. Hattab F, Al-Omari M, Angmar-Manson B, Daud N. The prevalence of nursing caries in one-to-four-year old children in Jordan. J Dent Childr 1999; Jan: 53-58.
62. Breastfeeding and Early Childhood Caries. (E.Petro, E.Hoxha, D.Kume, M.Kelmendi, D.Brovina), prezantim poster në 18-BASS Congress (Shkup, 2013).
63. Shiboski CH, Gansky SA, Ramos-Gomez F, Ngo L, Isman R, Pollick HF. The association of early childhood caries and race/ethnicity among California preschool children. J Public Health Dent 2003;63:38-46.
64. Davies GM, Blinkhorn FA, Duxbury JT. Caries among 3-year-olds in greater Manchester. Br Dent J 2001;190:381-384
65. Montero MJ, Douglass JM, Mathieu GM. Prevalence of dental caries and enamel defects in Connecticut head start children. Pediatr Dent 2003;25:235-239.
66. Stecksen-Blicks C, Sunnegardh K, Borssen E. Caries experience and background factors in 4-year-old children: time trends 1967-2002. Caries Res 2004;38:149-155.
67. Vanobbergen J, Martens L, Lesaffre E, Bogaerts K, Declerck D. Assessing risk indicators for dental caries in the primary dentition. Community Dent Oral Epidemiol 2001;29:424-434.
68. Lalloo R, Myburgh NG, Hobdell MH. Dental caries, socio-economic development and national oral health policies. Int Dent J 1999; 49(4): 196-202.
69. Davies GN. Early childhood caries – a synopsis. Comm Dent Oral Epidemiol 1998; 26(Supplement 1): 106-116.
70. Burt BA. Concepts of risk in dental public health. Community Dent Oral Epidemiol 2005;33:240-247.
71. Reisine ST, Psoter W. Socioeconomic status and selected behavioral determinants as risk factors for dental caries. J Dent Educ 2001;65:1009-1016.
72. Chen M, Andersen RM, Barmes DE, Lerlercq MH, Little IS. Comparing oral health care systems. Geneva:WHO 1997. pp:149-164, 293-323.
73. Petersen PE. Sociobehavioural risk factors in dental caries, international perspectives. Community Dent Oral Epidemiol 2005;33:274-279.
74. Psoter WJ, Pendrys DG, Morse DE, Zhang H, Mayne ST. Associations of ethnicity/race and socioeconomic status with early childhood caries patterns. J Public Health Dent 2006; 66(1): 23-9.
75. Kiwanuka SN, Astrom AN, Trovik TA. Dental caries experience and its relationship to social and behavioural factors among 3-5 year-old children in Uganda. Int J Paediatr Dent 2004; 14(5): 336-46.
76. Sheiham A, Watt RG. The common risk factor approach: a rational basis for promoting oral health. Community Dent Oral Epidemiol 2000;28:399-406.
77. Ribeiro NM, Ribeiro MA. Breastfeeding and early childhood caries: a critical review. J Pediatr (Rio J) 2004;80:S199-S210.
78. Mahejabeen R, Sudha P, Kulkarni SS, Anegurdi R. Dental caries prevalence among preschool children of Hubli: Dharwad City. J. Indian Soc Pedod Prev Dent 2006; 24(1): 19-22.

79. Mattila M, Rautava P, Sillanpaá M, Paunio P. Caries in five-year-old children and associations with family-related factors. J Dent Res 2000; 79(3): 875-881.
80. Horowitz AM. Response to Weinstein: Public health issues in early childhood caries. Comm Dent Oral Epidemiol 1998; 26(Supplement 1): 91-95.
81. Inglehart M, Tedesco LA. Behavioral research related to oral hygiene practices: a new Gratrix D, Taylor GO, Lennon MA. Mothers' dental attendance patterns and their children's dental attendance and dental health. Br Dent J 1990;168:441-443.
82. century model of oral health promotion. Periodontol 2000 1995;8:15-23.
83. Daly B, Watt RG, Batchelor P, Treasure ET. Essential Dental Public Health. Oxford: Oxford University Press 2002. pp:47-61, 153-166.
84. Pine CM, McGoldrick PM, Burnside G, Curnow MM, Chesters RK, Nicholson J,Huntington E. An intervention programme to establish regular toothbrushing: understanding parents' beliefs and motivating children. Int Dent J 2000; 312-323.
85. Paunio P. Dental health habits of young families from South-Western Finland. Community Dent Oral Epidemiol 1994;22:36-40.
86. Petersen PE. Inequalities in oral health: the social contex for oral health. In: Pine CM, Harris R (eds). Community Oral Health. Berlin: Quintessence 2007. pp:31-58
87. Okada M, Kawamura M, Kaihara Y, Matsuzaki Y, Kuwahara S, Ishidori H, Miura K. Influence of parents' oral health behaviour on oral health status of their school children: an exploratory study employing a causal modelling technique. Int J Paediatr Dent 2002;12:101-108.
88. Hoxha E, Petro E, Brovina D, Kelmendi A. First dental visit in Albania. 2009; OP: 14-BaSS Congress.
89. Gussy MG, Waters EG, Walsh O, Kilpatrick NM. Early childhood caries: current evidence for aetiology and prevention. J Paediatr Child Health 2006;42:37-43.
90. Chan SC, Tsai JS, King NM. Feeding and oral hygiene habits of preschool children in Hong Kong and their caregivers' dental knowledge and attitudes. Int J Paediatr Dent 2002;12:322-331.
91. Petro E, Hoxha E, Kelmendi E. Dietary Habits of ECC in Albania. 2010;OP:15-BaSS Congress.
92. PetroE, Hoxha E, Brovina D, Kume D. Vlerësimi i lidhjes midis indeksit HEI dhe kariesit të femijerisë së hershme. 2011; referim ne Kongresin II-të Ndërkombëtar të Stomatologjisë.
93. Petro E, Hoxha E, Brovina E, Kume D. Kariesi i fëmijerisë së hershme, ndikimi dhe përcaktimi i dietes në ecurinë e tij. 2010; referim në Konferencën XVI Kombëtare Dentare Shqiptare.
94. Petro E, Hoxha E, Kelmendi M, Brovina D. Assessing the relationship between HEI index and Early Childhood Caries. Bulletin of Medicine Sciences. 2013;1:55-60.
95. Welbury R, Duggal M, Hosey M. Paediatric Dentistry - Third Edition 2005;8: 107-203.
96. American Dental Association (ADA). ADA statements on early childhood caries.2007.
97. American Association of Pediatric Dentistry (AAPD). Dental care for your baby. 2007.
98. Twetman S, Garcia-Godoy F, Goepferd SJ. Infant oral health. Dent Clin North Am 2000;44:487-505.
99. Edelstein B. Policy issues in early childhood caries. Comm Dent Oral Epidemiol 1998; 86-103.

100. Schroth RJ, Moffatt ME. Determinants of early childhood caries in rural Mantoba community: a pilot study. Pediatr Dent 2005; 27(2): 114-20.
101. Van Wyk PJ, Louw AJ, Du Plessi JB. Caries status and treatment needs in South Africa: Report of the 1999-2002 National Children's Oral health Survey. SADJ 2004; 59(6): 238-242.
102. Lopez-Del-Valle L, Velazquez-Quintana Y, Weinstein P, Domoto P, Le Roux B. Early childhood caries and risk factors in rural Puerto Rican children. J Dent Childr 1998; 65(2): 132-135.
103. Weinstein P. Public health issues in early childhood caries. Community Dent Oral Epidemiol 1998;26(1 Suppl):84-90.
104. O'Sullivan DM, Douglass JM, Champany R, Eberling S, Tetrev S, Tinanoff N. Dental caries prevalence and treatment among Navajo preschool children. J Public Health Dent 1994 ;54:139-144.
105. E.Petro, E.Hoxha, D.Brovina, D.Kume. Trajtimi endodontik i ndërlikimeve të kariesit të fëmijërisë së hershme. Revista Stomatologjike Shqiptare 2010; 2: 11-14.
106. Whelton H, O'Mullane DM. Public health aspects of oral diseases and disorders. Community Oral Health 1997; 6: 75-81.
107. Rose G. Sick individuals and sick populations. Int J Epidemiol 2001;30:427-432.
108. Burt BA. Prevention policies in the light of the changed distribution of dental caries. Acta Odontol Scand 1998;56:179-186.
109. Seppä L. The future of preventive programs in countries with different systems for dental care. Caries Res 2001;35(1 Suppl):26-29.
110. Featherstone JD. The continuum of dental caries, evidence for a dynamic disease process. J Dent Res 2004;83(Spec No C):C39-C42.
111. Ismail AI. Prevention of early childhood caries. Community Dent Oral Epidemiol 1998;26(1 Suppl):49-61.
112. Overton Dickinson A. Community oral health education. In: Mason J (ed). Concepts in Dental Public Health. Philadelphia: Lippincott Williams & Wilkin 2005. pp:139-157.
113. Rugg-Gunn AJ (ed). Sugarless towards the year 2000. Royal Society of Chemistry, 1994.
114. Rugg-Gunn AJ, Hackett AF, Appleton DR, Jenkins GN, Eastoe JE. Relationship between dietary habits and caries increment assessed over two years in 405 English adolescent schoolchildren. Arch Oral Biol 1984;29:983-992.
115. Featherstone JD. Delivery challenges for fluoride, chlorhexidine and xylitol. BMC Oral Health 2006;6(1 Suppl):S8.
116. Kowash MB, Pinfield A, Smith J, Curzon ME. Effectiveness on oral health of a long-term health education programme for mothers with young children. Br Dent J 2000;188:201-205.
117. Ripa LW. Nursing habits and dental decay in infants: "Nursing bottle caries". J Dent Childr 1978; Jul/Aug.
118. Febres C, Echeverri EA, Keene HJ. Parental awareness, habits, and social factors and their relationship to baby bottle tooth decay. Pediatr Dent 1997; 19(1): 22-27.
119. Milgrom P. Response to Reisine E Douglas: Psychological and behavioral issues in early childhood caries. Comm Dent Oral Epidemiol 1998; 26(Supplement 1): 45-48.
120. Newbrun E. Effectiveness of water fluoridation. J Public Health Dent 1989;49:279-289. Evans DJ, Rugg-Gunn AJ, Tabari ED, Butler T. The effect of fluoridation and social class on caries experience in 5-year-old Newcastle children in 1994

121. Evans DJ, Rugg-Gunn AJ, Tabari ED, Butler T. The effect of fluoridation and social class on caries experience in 5-year-old Newcastle children in 1994 compared with results over the previous 18 years. Community Dent Health 1996;13:5-10.
122. Jones S, Burt BA, Petersen PE, Lennon MA. The effective use of fluorides in public health. Bull World Health Organ 2005;83:670-676.
123. Twetman S. Prevention of Early Childhood Caries (ECC): Review of literature published 1998-2007. Eur Archs Paediatr Dent 2008;9:12-18.
124. Douglass JM, Douglass AB, Silk HJ. A practical guide to infant oral health. Am Fam Physician 2004;70:2113-2120.
125. Samadzadeh H, Bayat F. Dentists and obligatory public health service. Tehran: Ministry of Health and Medical Education, Oral Health Bureau 1999.
126. Kay E, Locker D. A systematic review of the effectiveness of health promotion aimed at improving oral health. Community Dent Health 1998;15:132-144.
127. Kay EJ, Locker D. Is dental health education effective? A systematic review of current evidence. Community Dent Oral Epidemiol 1996;24:231-235.
128. Nurko C, Skur P, Brown JP. Caries prevalence of children in an infant oral health educational program at a WIC clinic. J Dent Child (Chic) 2003;70:231-234.
129. Rong WS, Bian JY, Wang WJ, Wang JD. Effectiveness of an oral health education and caries prevention program in kindergartens in China. Community Dent Oral Epidemiol 2003;31:412-416.
130. American Association of Pediatric Dentistry (AAPD). Early childhood caries: unique challenges and treatment options. Pediatr Dent 2000;22:21.
131. Cohen LA, Horowitz AM. Community-based sealant programs in the United States: results of a survey. J Public Health Dent1993;53(4):241-245.
132. Petro E, Hoxha E, Ciko E. Efikasiteti i aplikimit të silanteve në parandalimin e ECC. 2012; referim në Konferencën II të SHSHPP.
133. Abramson JH (2014). Computer Programs for Epidemiologists: WIN-PEPI, version 11.43. http://www.brixtonhealth.com/pepi4windows.html
134. Quinonez RB, Keels MA, Vann Jr WF, Mclver FT, Heller K. Early childhood caries: Analysis of psychological and biological factors in a high-risk population. Caries Res 2001;35:376-383.
135. Pine et al., International comparisons of health inequalities in childhood dental caries. Community Dent Health 2004;21(1 Suppl):121-130.
136. Tseveenjav B. Preventive dentistry in Mongolia. PhD thesis, University of Helsinki, Finland. Helsinki: Yliopistopaino, 2004. Available at http://ethesis.helsinki.fi/julkaisut/laa/hamma/vk/tseveenjav/
137. Hallett KB, O'Rourke PK. Early childhood caries and infant feeding practice. Community Dent Health 2002;19:237-242.
138. Landis JR, Koch GG. The measurement of observer agreement for categorical data. Biometrics 1977;33:159-74.
139. Burazeri G, Roshi E. Metodologjia e kerkimit shkencor ne shendetin publik 2010; 4:79-87.
140. Fung MHT, Wong MCM, Lo ECM, CH Chu. Early Childhood Caries: A Literature Review. Oral Hyg Health 2013; 1:1-7.
141. Begzati-Rexhepi A, Begzati A, Dibrani N, Rexha L. The prevalence of ECC in preschool children in the Municipality of Kastriot, Kosovo. 2012; PP:17-BaSS Congress.

142. Hattab FN, Al-Omari MA, Angmar-Mansson B, Daoud N. The prevalence of nursing caries in one-to-four-year-old children in Jordan. ASDC J Dent Child 1999;66:53-58.
143. King NM, Wu IIM, Tsai JSJ. Caries prevalence and distribution, and oral health habits of zero- to four-year-old children in Macau, China. J Dent Child 2003;70:243-249.
144. Chu CH, Fung DS, Lo EC. Dental caries status of preschool children in Hong Kong. Br Dent J 1999;187:616-620.
145. WHO, Guidelines for mothers of lowbirth weight children, 2004.
146. Paunio P, Rautava P, Helenius H, Alanen P, Sillanpää M. The Finnish family competence study: The relationship between caries, Dental health habits and general health in 3-year-old Finnish children. Caries Res 1993;27:154-160.
147. Marques APF, Messer LB. Nutrient intake and dental caries in the primary dentition. Pediatr Dent 1992; 14:314-321.
148. King NM, Wei SHY. Nutrient, diet and dental health. J Human Nut 1986; 8(3):1679-1687.
149. Shulman JD. Is there an association between low birth weight and caries in the primary dentition? Caries Res, 2005; 39:161-167.
150. Lay PY, Seow WK, Tudehope DI, Rogers Y. Enamel hypoplasia and dental caries in very low birth weight children: a case-controlled, longitudinal study. Pediatr Dent 1997;19:42-49.
151. Peretz B, Kafka I. Baby bottle tooth decay and complications during pregnancy and delivery. Pediatr Dent 1997;19(1):34-37.
152. World Health Organization (WHO). Guiding principles for complementary feeding of the breastfed-child. Geneva: WHO 2003b.
153. Roberts GJ, Cleaton-Jones PE, Fatti LP, Richardson BD, Sinwel RE, Hargreaves JA, Williams S. Patterns of breast and bottle feeding and their association with dental caries in 1- to 4-year-old South African children. 1. Dental caries prevalence and experience. Community Dent Health 1993;10:405-413.
154. Hinds K, Gregory JR. National diet and nutrition survey: children aged 1½ to 4½ years. Vol 2: Report of the dental survey. London: HMSO 1995.
155. Unkel JH, Sanford JP, Hobbs G, Frere CL. Toothbrushing ability is related to age in children. J Dent for Children 1995; Sept-Oct: 346-348.
156. Widmer R. The first dental visit: an Australian perspective. Int J Paediatr Dent 2003;13:270.
157. Rayner JA. The first dental visit: A UK viewpoint. Int J Paediatr Dent 2003;13:269.
158. Nainar SM, Straffon LH. Targeting of Year One dental visit for United States children. Int J Paediatr Dent 2003;13:258-63.
159. Douglass JM, Douglass AB. Infant oral health education for pediatric and family practice residents. Pediatr Dent 2005;27:4
160. Weinstein P, Domoto P, Koday M, Leroux B. Results of a promising open trial to prevent baby bottle tooth decay: a fluoride varnish study. ASDC J Dent Child 1994;61:338-341.
161. Wang NJ. Caries preventative methods in child dental care reported by dental hygienists, Norway, 1995 and 2004. Actu Odontol Scand 2005; 63(6): 330-4.
162. Marinho VC, Higgins JP, Sheiham A, Logan S. Combinations of topical fluoride (toothpastes, mouthrinses, gels, varnishes) versus single topical fluoride for preventing dental caries in children and adolescents. Cochrane Database System Rev. 2004. Comment in: Evid Based Dent 2004; 5(2): 38.

163. Shellis RP, Duckworth RM. Studies on the cariostatic mechanisms of fluoride. Int Dent Journal 1994; 44: 263-273.
164. Center for Disease Control (CDC). Recommendations for using fluoride to prevent and control dental caries in the United States. Centers for Disease Control and Prevention. MMWR Recomm Rep 2001;17;50:1-42.
165. Schroth RJ, Moore P, Brothwell DJ. Prevalence of Early Childhood Caries in 4 Manitoba Communities. JCDA 2005; 71(8).
166. Schroth RJ, Smith PJ, Whalen JC, Lekic C, Moffatt ME. Prevalence of caries among pre-school children in north Manitoba. J Can Dent Assoc 2005; 71(1): 27.
167. Tinanoff N. The early childhood caries conference, 18-19 October 1997. Pediatr Dent 1997; 19: 8.
168. Tinanoff N. Association of diet with dental caries in preschool children. Dent Clin North Am 2005; 49(4): 725-37.
169. Tinanoff N, Kaste LM, Corbin SB. Early childhood caries: positive beginning. Comm Dent Oral Epidemiol 1998; 26(Supplement 1): 117-119.
170. Davies GM, Blinkhorn FA, Duxbury JT. Caries among 3-year-olds in greater Manchester. Br Dent J 2001;190:381-384.
171. Wendt LK, Hallonsten AL, Koch G. Dental caries in one- and two-year-old children living in Sweden. Part I - A longitudinal study. Swed Dent J 1991;15:1-6.
172. Schroder U, Widenheim J, Peyron M, Hagg E. Prediction of caries in 1 1/2-year-old children. Swed Dent J 1994;18:95-104.
173. Lopez Del Valle L, Velazquez-Quintana Y, Weinstein P, Domoto P, Leroux B. Early childhood caries and risk factors in rural Puerto Rican children. ASDC J Dent Child 1998;65:132-135.
174. Hallonsten AL, Wendt LK, Mejàre I, Birkhed D, Håkansson C, Lindvall AM, Edwardsson S, Koch G. Dental caries and prolonged breast-feeding in 18-month-old Swedish children. Int J Paediatr Dent 1995;5:149-155.
175. Grindefjord M, Dahllof G, Modeer T. Caries development in children from 2.5 to 3.5 years of age: a longitudinalstudy. Caries Res 1995;29:449-454.
176. Alaluusua S, Malmivirta R. Early plaque accumulation, a sign for caries risk in young children. Community Dent Oral Epidemiol 1994;22:273-276.
177. Tsubouchi J, Higashi T, Shimono T, Domoto PK, Weinstein P. A study of baby bottle tooth decay and risk factors for 18-month old infants in rural Japan. ASDC J Dent Child 1994;61:293-298.
178. Vachirarojpisan T, Shinada K, Kawaguchi Y, Laungwechakan P, Somkote T, Detsomboonrat P. Early childhood caries in children aged 6-19 months. Community Dent Oral Epidemiol 2004;32:133-142.
179. Wendt LK, Carlsson E, Hallonsten AL, Birkhed D. Early dental caries risk assessment and prevention in pre-school children: evaluation of a new strategy for dental care in a field study. Acta Odontol Scand 2001;59:261-266.
180. Weinstein P, Harrison R, Benton T. Motivating parents to prevent caries in their young children: one-year findings. J Am Dent Assoc 2004;135:731-738.
181. Dye BA, Shenkin JD, Ogden CL, Marshall TA, Levy SM, Kanellis MJ. The relationship between healthful eating practices and dental caries in children aged 2-5 years in the United States, 1988-1994. J Am Dent Assoc 2004;135:55-66.
182. Ayhan H. Influencing factors of nursing caries. J Clin Pediatr Dent 1996; 20(4): 313-315.

9. ANNEX

a) Structured questionnaire.

Please fill out the questionnaire by marking the right answer with X

1. Child's name_____ _____

2. Mother/Guardian name   Phone no.

3. Mother/Guardian education

Elementary ——————

Middle school ——————

High school ——————

College ——————

Post-graduate ——————

4. Income level: Compared to other Albanian families, do you think your family has an income level:

Lower ——————

About same ——————

Higher ——————

5. Child's birth weight

Under 2500 gr ——————

Over 2500 gr ——————

6. Has the child suffered any chronic disease?

Yes ——   name of disease _____

No ——

7. Has the child received any regular medication/treatment?

Yes ——   name of medication/treatment _____

No ——

8. Has the child received/receives any supplements?   Yes ⌷   No ⌷

Fluoride ——————

Calcium ——————

Iron ——————

Vitamins ——————

Other ——————   name _____

9. Child feeding methods

Natural, breast milk only ——————

Artificial, formula only ——————

Combination of both ——————

10. Did you stop breastfeeding after the age 1?   Yes ⌷   N o ⌷

11. Did the child take the bottle at night?   Yes ⌷   No ⌷

12. Bottle contents
Cow milk
Formula milk
Fruit juice
Tea
Others   name _____

13. Did you add sugar to the soothing bottle?   Yes   No

14. Did your child use the soothing bottle?   Yes   No

15. Did you coat the bottle with sugar or honey?   Yes   No

16. Age child started drinking from a cup _____

17. Age when child started eating solid foods _____

18. Does the child consume between meals food?   Yes ☐   No ☐

19. Does the child consume sugary products?   Yes ☐   No ☐

20. Does the child consume lollipops/sugared candies?   Yes ☐   No ☐

21. Does the child brush every day?   Yes ☐   No ☐

22. Age when your child started brushing teeth _____

23. How many times a day does your child brush?
Once a day
Twice a day
More than twice

24. Does your child brush before bed?   Yes ☐   No ☐

25. Who brushes your child's teeth?
Child himself
Parent/guardian
Child under parent supervision

26. Age child first visited dentist's office _____

27. Does your child have regular dental check-ups?   Yes ☐   No ☐

28. Does your child have sealants placed?   Yes ☐   No ☐

29. Did your child have fluoridation performed at dentist/kindergarten?   Yes ☐   No ☐

Thank you for your cooperation!

Dental File
Faculty of Dental Medicine
Department of Stomatological Therapy
Prevalence of early childhood caries in children 3-5 years old in Tirana

1. Serial number ☐ ☐ ☐ ☐

2. Date ☐ ☐   ☐ ☐   ☐ ☐ ☐ ☐

3. Kindergarten No. ☐ ☐

4. Child's name _____

5. Age in years ☐

6. Gender M/F ☐

7. Dental status according to WHO

55	54	53	52	51	61	62	63	64	65

85	84	83	82	81	71	72	73	74	75

A= no caries
B= with caries
C= filling with caries
D= filling without caries

E= extraction because of caries
F= sealant
T= trauma/fracture
- =cannot be examined

8. deft Index

dt _____
et _____
ft _____
deft _____

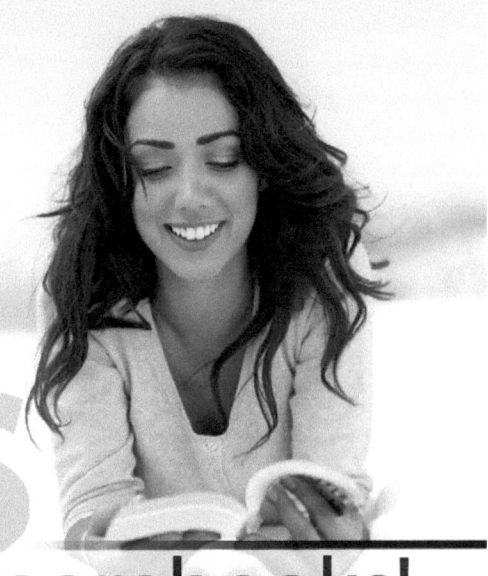 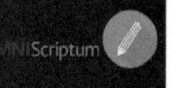

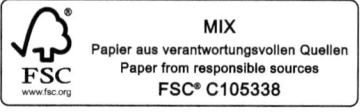